To Lawrence Huber
Thanks for all the hard
work
Marion R. Daney
_4-21-10_

LATEX IS NOT MY FRIEND

MARION RONEE DANEY
PHARMACY TECHNICIAN

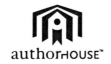

authorHOUSE™

1663 LIBERTY DRIVE, SUITE 200
BLOOMINGTON, INDIANA 47403
(800) 839-8640
WWW.AUTHORHOUSE.COM

First published by AuthorHouse 12/20/05

ISBN: 1-4208-9430-7 (sc)

Library of Congress Control Number: 2005909985

Printed in the United States of America
Bloomington, Indiana

This book is printed on acid-free paper.

CONTENTS

ACKNOWLEDGE

Most of all I like to Thank Yahweh (Lord) for choosing me to do the Great Task that he bestows upon me. I pray that I am humble servant so that I can allow the Glory of Elohim (God) shine through always. Since my Nightmare with latex beginning, I trusted in the Yahshua (Holy Spirit) to give me strength and hope and most of all Faith that I would survive. When Yahshua (Holy Spirit) spoke to me and told me to write about latex. I said to myself why me? I knew in my heart, I was going to do something great. I have been writing poetry for years and the poems were beautiful. I knew that it was a great spirit giving me the words of Wisdom. I knew it was a reason why I wrote so well. I did not think anything about it. Therefore, Yahshua (Holy Spirit) took me from knowing nothing about latex to knowing and guiding me to all the information, I needed to complete this book. At times, I was driven and I did not know what was going on. I had a horrific experience with latex and by my research; I realized that I was not alone. I know that this is my Destiny and I must step into the footsteps that are in front of me. Sometimes the night was so dark that the light could not penetrate, and now I had to face Fear and strand straight up for people that could not have a Voice that could be heard. Fear not because Yahshua (Holy Spirit) was with me through all my battles. I am honored and "His Will", will be done with Love, Integrity and Beauty will be in every word.

To my Darling son Jonathan, I love very much. I am so proud of you for being a great encouragement and strength in my life. I am proud to be your Mother. I know that at times I was not myself because of the horrific experience that I had to endure. Thanks for not giving up on me as a Mother. Thanks for your patients and understanding.

To my Father (who has passed on) and my Mother, I am grateful for all the support and Love that you gave me. You were always there for my son Jonathan through all the rough roads that I had to endure. I know that my father is looking down at me from heaven and he is smiling. Your Love had given me strength and Integrity to stand up for what is right. I Love you.

Thanks to my sisters April and Margo for always is being there. I Love both of you.

To a Friend whom I have always called her my Vanilla Sister, Toni Velasquez. Even though we have had our difference and a Slap Down Fist-Fight, some how we seemed to continue to be friends.

For my Spiritual Friend Virdell, for always listening to my tears and hear my pain. Our Spiritual conversations had kept me focus on what I must endure. I have to stay true to my Destiny. Because that is who I am. Love.

For a Special Friend Jatawn, that lives in Louisiana. Thanks for always listening to me even though you are far always you have always been there. Your encouragements through my rough times and just want to thank you for being there. I love you.

For my Uncle Larry & Aunt Joye Jackson Thanks for being they are for my son Jonathan and me. When were first having allergic reactions at work because of the latex? You both were there for me and Uncle Larry tried to fine me a doctor. Thanks so much for being there for your understanding and love. I love you both very much.

This thanks is for a Special Friend, Mr. Fred Fischer. Who was like a Grandpa to my son, and took Jonathan under his wings and loved him. He taught my son many important things about life. Gramps also showed Jonathan how important good values are. Jonathan and Fred were like Buddies; Jonathan drove Fred to the store, and Doctor Offices they always were together. His whole family embrace Jonathan and I, and made us part of their family. We miss him terribly since he is now with the Angels. Thanks to his family Julie and John Amrhein and Larry Fischer.

PREFACE

My intention on writing this book is to give information and experiences about latex allergies. By no means, do I intend to offend anyone or company who produce any products that contain latex. While reading this book on the subject latex allergies do not panic. There has been problems with latex gloves as well as other latex products; a lot of them have been changed to benefit everyone.

Since 1996, I have suffered with latex allergies. I developed Asthma and began experiencing periods of deep depressions. Due to the severe reactions that I was experiencing my last employment date was November 4, 1996. I developed rash, Asthma and began experiencing periods of deep depression. I started research 1997, because I feel as though this was more that

Psychosomatic. When my job stops, paying me I was so appalled, this was not my fault the allergy that I have developed while working. I said to myself I would write a story and send it to Medical Journal. I was so angry and hurt I felt so deceived. This little voice inside of me said that if you do things out of angry nothing good will come of it. I wanted to tell everything! So now, I know it was the Heavenly Father speaking to me. He led me to write my story, gather up information on latex allergies, and put together as a book. I said to him do you know whom you are talking to? I have never written a book before and I do not even know where to start. I have been writing poetry since I was 17 years old. I had felt that deep inside my heart that the poetry that I was led to write, it was just a beginning of a greater purpose. So I humbled myself and said a prayer, "help me Father in Heaven show me what you want me do." I will be obedient and carry out your will Father. I realized that this is my Destiny and I was born to write. Therefore, I continued to do my research on latex allergy. I did not know how to do research because, I never researched any subjects before, I was only hoping that it was correct. I continued to gather up information from the Medical Journals and Internet sites for my book. I did not know how long the research would take me, to complete the book. I felt inside of me that my book was coming to an end. I realized that I learned a lot about latex allergies, and I was not alone in my suffering. I know that latex allergy affects people all over the world. I saw that this problem dealing with latex allergy opened up the Medical field eyes. The doctors, scientist, and legislators had to do something to resolve some problems that latex has caused. You will see in this book how hard everyone worked together to figure out how latex allergies started. Latex gloves, is designed to protect everyone from diseases, infections, etc. At the same, it was creating an allergy. First of all the doctors and nurses were the first victims because, the medical professions were required to wear gloves, and the were made from latex. They did not think they were creating a problem. Until, the doctors, nurses and other medical staff started having problems. Some of the Medical staff were in jeopardy and interrupted their careers as result of this allergy. Latex gloves were sensitizing some of the Doctors, Nurses and some did have anaphylactic reactions. The Dental offices were experiencing some of the same reactions to latex gloves and products that contained latex. The problems were occurring, because the medical professions use numerous gloves a day. The powder in the gloves are cornstarch this helped the doctors and nurses putting glove on and off easier. What happen was the powder bond with the allergens in the gloves, so when the gloves taken off the particles became airborne. So when latex became airborne the Medical Staff then inhaled the particles. That is why some people developed Asthma, dermatitis, and some became sensitized to latex. When these problems occurred, there were limited amounts of information available and a few Doctors understood this allergy. Many people were baffled and even today they still trying to understand the whole Latex Allergy. The Food and Drug Administration received many reports about Latex Glove Allergies. The FDA had to investigate these reports plus reports of deaths that occurred as result of latex exposure. It seems as though the more a person would wear latex gloves, that individual sometimes became sensitized. The Doctors noticed that children having numerous surgeries like spinal bifida, they were going into Anaphylactic Shock while in surgery. Even some adults having numerous surgeries were having anaphylactic reactions and some doctors thought they were having reactions from the medications. There are tests for latex allergies available in the Allergist Office. People that are allergic to latex, there are some fruits that have some of the same allergens that latex have. If you have, any reactions contact your doctor's office. Even a simple, blowing up a latex balloon a child can have a reaction. This has been a great learning experience for me and I am in a position to share my story. I hope that people will understand that they are not alone. In addition, I share with you my pain, angry, depression and emptiness. This was very difficult task for me to continue to write this book. I realized that I could not walk away from my Destiny.   Destiny presented herself to me, I was afraid and shaking but I continued my journey. I stepped into shoes that she put before me and I took one-step at a time. If I had denied Destiny, I would have then walked away from who I was to become   I had to allow Destiny Greatness and Wisdom to show me the way. I totally opened up myself to the Universe, and I realized it was Magical. The Universe opened up her arms and shared with me Kindness, Love, Mercy, and her Wisdom, which it became apart of me. The Universe gave me all I needed to complete the book, "Latex Is Not My Friend."

THE PEOPLE
WHO INSPIRITED ME

When I of think Lieutenant John, from the Navy officer, who stood up to make awareness of the problems of latex. I admired him, but in the progress of his goal, he died in the hospital from complication from latex allergy. I am grateful and I wonder why my life was spared. However, his voice will be heard. I hear a story of Lance Armstrong, he fought against the disease cancer and won the battle. He is a cyclist and he won Tour de France race 7 times in a role. The strength and courage beyond his mind made him triumph more than anyone else. I look at Oprah Show and watch from where she came and now. What a different contributions she has made in her life. She is very inspirational all over the world. I admire her stadium, courage, and most of all she had found love. The Love is an important tool in her life, which is her Richness beyond words that could ever speak. I look at a Motivation Speaker, Wayne Dwyer. His stories he lived in foster care and separated form his siblings. He continued his education with a degree. He speaks all over the world. He says we all come from a source. He has ability to make our own lives happier, stronger, and full of love if we choose. One thing I learned from him that I play over in mind many times. This was from a book "Intentions", what is your true intention when you do or stay anything? I know that the book was a gift to me from Divine Power and Wisdom it will do well. Because my Intentions are only to help people understand Latex Allergy, so they can protect themselves. Then they will understand and realize that they will not have to live in fear of latex. The people will know that the Companies that have made the products form latex, have stepped up to the plate and recognized and accepted the issues of the people. The Companies have made good decisions in making their product safe.

This was to protect the people. Creflo Dollar is a Minister for "Changing your World", he preached on how the Holy Spirit chooses people to carry out his will. Holy Spirit can choose someone that knows nothing about a subject and guild them teaching them all they need to know. Your break through is right around the corner. Joyce Meyer preaches on Double for your Trouble, when you have suffered through a lot in your life your Heavenly Father will bless you. You have to have faith, you have to stay strong, and believe that every thing works together for good that love Yahweh (God). TD Jakes preaches on you have to think outside of the box.

Some movies have given me hope. One in particular is the Last Samurai with Tom Cruise. I see Loyal, Respect, Integrity, and most of Honor. Sometimes I feel like a Warrior and I have the duty to stand up with Integrity and with Honor. I have been chosen to do Greatness in my life and I have stand Tall. I he captive in land he knew not. He learned the ways of the Samurai. He realized that the people were have to use all of my Faith that I have acquired in my spirit to do what My Destiny has put before me. I will tell the stories to make sure that their Voices be heard. All the Doctors and Scientist work was not in Vain. These Latex problems were all over the county and so many of the professionals, would not lye down and do nothing. They stood up and demanded changes. Troy the movie was an impact on me, watching it. It was overwhelming and powerful. The Warrior planed by Brad Pitt was amazing as he was Achilles that led the Greek army against the Kingdom of Troy. Achilles was strong and made to fight and be a Warrior. He seems as though he was invisible. He wanted his name go on forever. The courage that he possessed and the respect of the soldiers it was breath taking. In this world, you must stand up for something and have a great will to achieve Victory. The Universe Constance reminds me to take all of who I am what the Universe shows me that I am a Warrior. One thing that Achilles seems to see part of him knew Loving someone gave him peace in a time of War. I watched another extraordinary true story Hidalgo. An American cowboy and his mixed breed Pure Mustang (Untamed) horse compete against the world's greatest Arabian horses 100 in the dangerous "Ocean of Fire" race! Greatest endurance race all times Viggo Mortensen plays this part of Frank Hopkins the cowboy, this movie was built from great character integrity, courage, love, and for someone that was lost he found his true Destiny. He risk his life to save a princess not realizing that he was saving his self for a greater purpose He loved the Mustang horses and on land which he had lived Mustang can run free. Than we know or understand why we are lead, to do what Government plan to gather up the Wild horses Mustangs know it day and the government wanted to destroy the horses. He even let his horse be free to run with the other Mustangs. I realize that sometimes we are chosen, for a greater purpose. He even let his horse be free so he could run with the other Mustangs. His purpose from the money he won from the race he able to purchase the land so the Wild Horses run free and be free. I realize that sometimes we are chosen for a greater purpose, which we do not always understand at the time. A force con captivate you and pull you in and give you courage strength, integrity Frank Hopkins had these qualities inside of him. He was able to learn to have Faith in himself to do something extraordinary for the Greater good.

One movie I watched touched my heart for so many years was about saving Mountain Gorillas, "Gorillas in The Mist," The Adventure of Dian Fossey. This young woman was Dian Fossey and she was a Physical Therapist. These Mountain Gorillas became a part of soul and her passion and then her obsession. She scarified everything to save their lives and a place for them to live. She could not walk away from the gorillas, they became her family, and she laughed with them, played with them. At this time in Africa, these Mountain Gorillas were being Butchered and sold their hands and heads. At the far ends of the Earth, she found a reason to live, and a cause to fight for their lives. This was her destiny she embraced it with joy. She could not accept waking up every day and not seeing the Mountain Gorillas faces. Her live would have been empty.

THERE ARE ANGELS OF MERCY

I feel as though I have to acknowledge the people that have helped me through my Rain Storm.

Primarily, I like to thank the Doctors at The University of Michigan Health System. The first Doctor is Dr. Eileen M. Reickert, M.D., and she listened to my horror story. She understood all of my frustrations and concerns. At that moment I wanted to reach out and huge her. I felt as though she was saving my life. She stated that University of Michigan Hospital understands Latex Allergy and she stated that she was going to send me to the best Allergist. His name is Dr. Martin E. Hurwitz, M.D.; he is part of the University of Michigan Hospital. I meet Dr. Hurwitz and he listened and said my impression is that the patient probably has contact dermatitis sensitivity to latex or some component of processed latex. I think breathlessness and most of the respiratory difficulties are due to probably a combination on hyperventilation and vocal cord dysfunction syndrome. He suggested that I have referral to Dr. Norman Hogikyan, M.D. at University of Michigan Otolaryngology Voice Clinic in Livonia with perhaps a visit to Dr. Haxler, who is Speech Pathologist and could perhaps instruct the patient in techniques to keep glottis open on inspiration, would be worth while. Ms. Daney fits the profile of an individual who is likely to suffer from Paradoxical Vocal Cord Closure. I was relieved finally; someone really understood my reactions the Latex gloves. He explained when I had bad reaction and I broke out in hives across my back, chest, and shoulders. I just keep thinking this doctor is my last hope, if he did not understand I was going to committee my self, just lock me up and put a straight jacket on me. I felt the Psyche Ward was going to get another patient, because here I come. I am glad it did work out for me. I went to clinic and took tests, one I had swallow a tube camera up through noise and it had to go down my throat. It reached down to Bronchitis Tubes to see my where my breathing problems coming from and check for damages. I took up some speech therapy sessions. I was singing "Mary Had a Little Lamb," and walking up and down the hallways talking. This was difficult for me because, I Do not have the ability to walk and talk at the same time. I also like to thank Dr. Joel. Heidelbaugh, M.D. and especially thanks to Dr. Eileen Reichert, M. D., and because of her I was able to get my Disability.

I like to acknowledge my doctors at that work at Family First Clinic that is association with Mount Clements Hospital. I knew at this time that many doctors were not very knowledgeable about Latex. I was forced to change doctors because of insurance reasons. These doctors were patient, understanding, and they listened to me. I was grateful to the doctors who were, Dr. Christopher M. O'Connell. D. O, Dr. Kristin Beougher, D.O., Dr. Loren De Carlo, D.O. Also, I like to give a special thanks to Kathy and D'andra who work in the same doctors' office. They are Medical Assistances that were very kind and understanding to me. I appreciated that they were compassionate and kind. I had to go to Pulmonary & Critical Care Associates, P. C., which was located in St Clair Shores. My Doctor is Dr. Christopher W. Hughes, M. D., F.C.C.P., his impression: History of Latex Allergy, Vocal Cord Dysfunction, History of Asthma with Multiple triggers He realized that I had a difficult time dealing with my Latex Allergy and Depression. He knew that Latex Allergy was complicated and a lot of the Medical Doctors had limited source of information on Latex. Understanding Latex Allergy was a great task. I shared some information on Latex Allergy to Dr. Christopher W. Hughes. I am grateful that Dr. Hughes is my doctor he is very humble, kind, and he always took time to listen to what I was saying.

I like to thank my two Lawyers: Mr. Terry Berlin and Mr. Ronald Applebaum.
If it were not for Mr. Terry Berlin dedication, I would not have received my Workmen's Compensation and Disability Benefits. For the case against the Latex Corporation that Mr. Ronald Applebaum it was dropped. The reason were because, the blood test (RAST TEST), which this test measurement the IgE Level in the Blood. My test was negative, even tough I had latex reactions while working and even going to ER for 2 ½ hours that was not enough. Even until this day I still suffer the same reactions that a person being exposure to Latex. The Courts put stimulation on the Latex cases, and some Latex Corporations stated no regulation on gloves and changing the

amounts of powder in Glover could compromise the standards of the gloves. There were a lot of Latex cases dropped in the Courts. I appreciated all of Mr. Ronald Applebaum's dedication and hard work I realized that it was not his fault that the case was dropped. It was beyond control.

There are Many Angel's of Mercy that I have encounter in my life. I am grateful and privilege to have been in their presences I know that my Heavenly Father Loves me so much he send all of the Angels to guide my footsteps.

Stand Up

When I had stopped work November 4, 1996 as a Pharmacy Technician, I was devastated Since, I went to school for Pharmacy Technician program for six months. What was going to become of me? In January 1997, I watched 20/20, this particular night Barbara Walters did a program on Latex. I was very shocked and I had never heard of any problems discussed concerns on Latex on TV before. Barbara Walter interviewed a man and his family. This was his story. His wife was allergic to latex, and she took Benadryl whenever she was exposed to latex. One day she went to hospital to visit her niece in OR Recovery unit after she had surgery. She stayed a while and did touch the hospital bed. She came home put 3 kids to bed and her husband was down stairs. She took a Benadryl and went to bed. Her husband came check on her to see how she was feeling, and he noticed that she was shortness of breath and turning blue. She rushed to the hospital, she was given medication to control allergic reaction. Her recovery was going fine, until she had been served her meal. One of the things she ate was a Banana. Later that evening she did not realize she had a reaction to banana, while she went to sleep that night. The next day nurses checked on her, the medical staff knew it was something terribly wrong. She was deprived of oxygen. She apparently when into Anaphylaxis Shock and ended up having a stroke. She had difficulty speaking, walking, and part of her body was affected. The hospital at that time was not aware that Banana has some of the same allergens that Latex have. The banana continued the reaction after she ate it just like the latex did her. She had to take a lot of rehabilitation to help her recovery. I know it was very difficult for her husband to take care of her and the small children. Unfortunately, Doctors and Nurses still did not understand Latex allergic reactions. Many medical staff also had been exposed to Latex and was having health problems. I feel although I am blessed that I did not eat a banana after I had an allergic reaction to latex. I was spared from that, and why? I know it was a Navy Officer Lieutenant Harold R. "Hal" Henderson, RN, BSN, CEN, and TNCC. NC USN/RET, 40, of San Diego, California. He was working with Elastic; this Company was set up to inform people about Latex exposure. The Lieutenant Harold R. Henderson was a Register Nurse and he worked in a hospital. He was having allergic reactions and he wanted so much to prevent other from having to go through same loss of career, health and self-esteem that he did. Associated with latex allergy. At that time, Latex was still being investigated. He did die from the result of respiratory and cardiac complications and suffered a massive heart attack. This sad day was August 27, 1997 I felt so badly for him and I must make sure his legacy lives. He stood for Integrity, Respect, and Loyalty, as a Soldier should. My heart cries for him, because he was trying to save people's lives and in the process, he lost his own. How heroic he was. I know it is my responsibility to carry on and stand up for this cause, I was chosen for. My heart is very heavy and I have a responsibility to keep valid information out there to protect the innocent. I will make sure that Lieutenant Harold R. Henderson voice will be heart; he did not die in Vain. One day I wish to visit his grave and tell him my story and my pain.

I was looking at the Regis & Kelly Show one day, this was about a year a 2004. Kelly Rippa was talking about an allergic reaction that she had. Kelly for some reason was going to us a hot tub. When she got into the hot tub, she noticed that she was itching some and it got worse. She got out and noticed she whelms appearing on her legs and the itching was unbearable. She had to go to doctor. She found out that the hot tub was made with different material and on was Latex. She said that she felt terrible and that this experience was horrible. The doctor prescribed medications for her allergeric reaction to latex.

WHAT HAS THE WHOLE EXPERIENCE TAUGHT ME?

Wow! When I think about the Latex Experience, I am overwhelmed. I realized that I had to open up my eyes and see the pain of others. My pain inside was so deep it was choking me and blinded me. I was then consumed in it. When my eye could see the truth, I could no longer deny my Destiny. I denied of Depressed for a while because I never knew about it. Depression is a world of its own. It can make you think of things and put thoughts in your in your mind, that you would never think about. I got to the point of wanting to harm others and myself. I had those thoughts and as I think of them, I am so ashamed of myself. How was it possible that something invaded that I am true to overcome my spirit. Who could possibly be that strong to take over me? I did not even fight it because. I did not even see it coming. Next thing I knew I was drowning and drowning. Lost in a place where hope, peace, love, and power did not exist. I was in a daze for so long that I do not even remember years that went by. It was a burr for me. I remembering sleeping long hours did not want to get out of the bed. Taking my son to school and the only thing I, thoughts were I could not wait to go back to bed. I did not make my bed any more even now I do not. I do not even have the desire to. Why should I am just going to get back in the bed. It was not a purpose for me. With all the medicines I was taking Benadryl, blood pressure, inhalers, and depression, at times I was drowsy and I could care less. I would cook sometimes then I would go lye down again. My son did not understand and I did not either realize what was happening to me. At time, I did feel better but most of the times, I was so heavenly burden. I was just like an empty shell. Hollow inside I could not hear my heart beating. I did not even think I had a heart anymore. I did not feel alive. I just existed in a Nightmare that seemed to pull all of the life in me out. Laughter seemed to be apart of my past. I did not enjoy TV programs. When I saw people, happy or good things would happen to people. It would make me sad and I would cry and cry. I felt I should be happy for them but I could not. My sorrows and grief was running through my total essence. I would feel down for days, it was, as I was on a roller coaster and I cold not getting off. I just kept going down. The medicine helped sometimes and sometime not. However, I had to stop watching some programs because it was just too hard. I could not bare the pain at times. Even until today, I have that problem. No, I realize that I have learned to be more patient, kind and have mercy on others. I am not the only one in pain in this world. If I can help others even with a kind word or a hug, I will do that. This book will open a door for me that I did not know what is on the other side. I with the grace of the Holy Spirit I know that I will be at a good place. .

Marion Ronee Daney

THIS IS A QUESTION THAT MY LAWYER ASKED ME TO ANSWER: THIS WAS MY RESPONSE.

17. State how your latex injury has affected you other than as relates to employment?

My nightmare is every day when I wake up in the morning. My life is hell. I cannot eat at times and cannot sleep. Ever time I go out I live in fear that I will have a bad reaction and I will not recover. Fumes, odors, perfumes, are everywhere even the road when work put asphalt down it is mixed with rubber (old tires) that make it hard to breath. I have reactions every day. When I go out in the environment shopping and driving. I always in center all these odors. Which it makes it difficult shopping I have to cover my mouth. `I hold my breath to try to limit a reactions but that is impossible. My reactions can last 3-5 days. When I cannot catch my breath, I have to lye down and use the Ventoin inhaler, and Benadryl does not prevent me fro having reactions. They can only help me after relations happens. That is what frightens me. The cold-cool-crisp air, hot air, air conditions, air driving trigger reactions and I have to keep my inhaler handy always with my epipen. When these reactions happen I get shortness of breath, lungs hurt with sharp pain in my chest areas, I have to hold my chest area, while walking I get shortness of breath, shortness of breath walking upstairs, I can't walk long distance without sitting down resting, I can't jogging, roller blade, run, play any sport that deal with any fast pace, ice skating, carrying packages to my door from car I have to rest and get out of breath. Some of the stores I go into I immediately have to leave because of all the perfumes, fragrances in the air my lungs hurt immediately, going to the public restrooms with eh deodorizes

8

in there I have to leave right after. I cannot take my son place because of the weather, odors and perfumes in the air. I get so depressed because he is a child and does not know why his mother cannot do things like she use too. When I think about latex and talk about it I hyperventilating, I get shortness of breath. I cannot sleep at night and I have anxiety attacks. I always worry about having a reaction I have Panic Disorder when I think about what this damn latex has done to y life I star crying, shaking, I can't concentration, I loose I perspective in my life, I don't care sometimes what happens to me, At times I want to hurt myself. If I cut my wrist will I bleed and how much, I have thoughts of driving of the bridge right into the lake and I won' have to think about latex ever again. I feel empty inside and empty, I feel like I am in a hole and I cannot get out I am totally trapped in a latex world. I do not clean up my home at times because I do not care; I have not life any more. It breaks my heart I cannot be normal and breathe again. Now because of the asthma, I have Vocal Cord Dysfunction Syndrome I cannot control my vocal cords, they close while I take at times and I get shortness of breath and the fumes, fragrant, cleaning products trigger that to happen. I constantly go back and forth to the doctors, which is difficult for me in any type of weather. Going to doctor office fragrances always around no matter what.

My emotions are so out of control at times when I think out it scream and just put me in a straight jacket and a padded room so I would not have any more pain. I cannot keep living like this it horrible to have so many restrictions. I would like to cut my risks and drive straight into the lake where I can have a peace of mind. I did not have a peace of mind anymore. I live in fear always follows me wherever I go. My life is so traumatize that I am not the same person. I lost who I am I have no life any more latex destroyed me.

Latex Is Not My Friend

Latex Allergy can be deadly like a bullet to one's heart. I know that some people do not take this situation seriously. Therefore, I will begin to elaborate on how my Nightmare began.

Hello! My name is Marion Ronee Daney, I am 36 years old, and I have a 10-year-old son. Starting over and living with my parents. Making a career decision, which was Pharmacy Technician Program at Academy Of Health Careers? This school would provide me with the experience and knowledge that I would use to establish my career in a hospital setting. September 1992 to May 1993, I completed my course and have a certificate of completion also included Intern shift. I worked a Perry Drugs story from October 1993 to July 1994. During May 1994, I landed a job at a Hospital as a Pharmacy Technician. During May 1994 until September, I learned the outpatient procedures and oral baby dosing system. The other part of September, I was trained the process of IV preparation. Learning Chemotherapy Hood and making Chemotherapy IV's that was the next step. During the process of making chemotherapy I would have to wear a 1) mask, 2) gown, 3) sterile latex gloves. I noticed that I started breaking out after I wore the gloves. I reported to Supervisor on duty Mr. Sims. Head said put some anti-biotic ointment on the rash. This occurred about three more times, it was a rash, it itched, and it was red. I showed him again and told the Head Supervisor. She did not say any thing about it. Therefore, I made a decision that I would use non-latex gloves. Which I ended up using plastic gloves (vinyl) under the sterile latex gloves and hopefully that would resolve the problem. No one suggested that I was or it was possible that I could be allergic to latex. Mr. Sims said that the gloves contain powder that is why you have been breaking out. No one ever questioned me from the supervisor if the problems continued and no mention at all. In May or June, the package of the latex gloves changed from green to blue the latex glove company. In the Pharmacy Department, we use these products daily. My shifts vary from one week to the next. I noticed that my nose would run more than usually, but I thought nothing of it. I have Hay fever during different parts of the year, so when the air on and the fan blowing constantly I thought it was normal. I noticed that my nose would run year around. The hospital has Same Day Surgery Floor, which I delivered Medical Pumps and supplies on the unit. In October 1996, I was to be trained for OR Pharmacy Satellite Unit. I noticed that I had runny nose more frequent, and I thought it was from the air blowing. During my training period, I would replace trays in the operating room, which consist of twenty trays. This procedure was done every morning before surgery began. On the fifth day working in OR Pharmacy, my training was complete. I notched that after delivering the trays around 10 am, my arms and legs started to itching some. I went to lunch at 12 am came back at 1pm. I noticed that the itching became little more. I said to Pharmacist on duty, Kerry said to me Marion you must be allergic to Latex. Kerry said Marion you must be allergic Latex, at 2:30 I left the OR Pharmacy. I went to the Coordinator, which was Ms. Li and I stated to her I was itching. She said for me to take Benadryl, she had no comment. I reported the incident to Ms. Janet the Supervisor, she act as if it was nothing. I even told her that Kerry said that I must be allergic to latex. I reported the incident to Ms. Vicki, the Director of Pharmacy, and she had no comment or suggestions. Both of management did not even suggest that I am latex sensitivity. On October 23, 1996, I worked in the morning in the IV room. I was required to do two Chemotherapy IVs. I gowned up, put my mask on and then put vinyl gloves on then latex gloves on top. This was at 10:00 am; I finished at 10:30. I noticed that at 10:45 my back started to itch a little. As time went on it got, worsen. I had my back against the corner walls and racks going up and down trying to relieve the itching. At 11:30am the Pharmacist on duty Ms. Martha suggest for me to take Benadryl 25 mg. The itching became unbearable! I went to the Supervisor she wrote me up a report, so I go to ER. My back was inflamed and I had broken out. At 12 am, the doctor examined my back. At 12:15, the nurse gave me Benadryl 50mg IM. I stayed in ER until 2:30pm. The doctor prescribed Prednisone 2mg Dose pack to be taken for 6 days. My mother had to put me up from the hospital ER, because I could not drive. Dr. Mamo, MD. Final Impressions: Acute Allergic Reaction, there was a rash on her back, shoulders, and neck. The next day I stayed home to rest my back. I called employed Health department to see if I can be tested for latex allergy. I talked to nurse Ruth, she suggested that I call Workmen's Compensation department. I called Workmen's Compensation department I talked with Tammy. I told her about my incident and going to ER. I told her that I needed to be tested for latex. Tammy told me that she could not help me. I told her this happened at work. Sorry I cannot help you. The next day I talked with my Director. I asked her what I was going to do about the situation. She said "Oh Marion do not worry about it or get upset. I pleaded with the Supervisor, Ms Janet, how am I going to resolve this problem Ms. Li the Coordinator approached me in the same office that I was, She said to me "Marion if you are allergic to latex it is very dangerous for you to be here. You must get another job. I did not understand what she was trying to stress to me. Later that day I went to personnel department and I talked to management, Ms. Carol. I showed her the papers from ER and she told me that if I can prove that I am allergic to latex. She could then remove me from my job. She gave me a phone number to help me resolve this matter. They would not pay for the latex test for me. This happened to me on the job, I was very disturbed. I did not know what I was up against. Latex my Nightmare, my Monster that was real for me and no one wanted to take time to help me. I explained to Ms. Carol that I had no insurance and there is no way I could pay for the test. Please can you help me? No one was listening. I called a hospital to make an appointment, so I could be tested. The only appointment they had was a month away. I told the receptionist; yeah about time I get there, I could be dead. I decided to call another hospital; they told me I needed a referral from my doctor to make an appointment with the Allergist. I was so upset. I called my Uncle Dr Larry Jackson, who is a Psychiatrist. I explained my situation to him. He could not understand why my job did not want to help me be tested. He tried to get leads on how I get some help on testing. At this time, I continued to work. I had to deliver Doctor's tray to Operating Unit, I talked to our Supervisor Martha. Within minutes I started itching all over my necks and arms I left out running out of the unit. On Sunday, I delivered IVs and supplies to four center. This is where they deliver babies. I was there about ten minutes. I continued the delivery to the rest of the units required. When I returned to the Pharmacy Department within a half-hour, I started itching all over my body. I reported to the Pharmacist on duty, Ms. Mang. I took a Benadryl 25mg when I got home. The next day I called ER and I talked to John an RN. He said call back employee health and talk to Mary. I did so, she sent me over to another hospital. My appointment was with a Physician Assistance her name was Susan Howard. She stated that it appears that you are allergic to latex, and she said that did you know that you could die from being exposed to latex. You will have to be limited at the workplace. You should avoid latex gloves, and patient care units, areas of the pharmacy for Chemotherapy reparation that is where latex gloves are more prevalent. She also told me that she was allergic to latex, her eyes would swell and parts of her face. Finally, someone understands about latex reactions. If you have to deliver to a unit on hospital floor do your work quickly and get out fast. Personnel Department gave me phone number to Disease Control and she if you can help you. On 11-4, I contacted Disease Control, Ms. Hope. The reason was to see if they could monitor the hospital for levels of latex. She stated that this situation beyond her. On 11-5, the Director of Pharmacy discussed my situation with me. She stated that I could not come back to work because she could not promise me a latex free environment. I could not have restrictions working in Pharmacy Department. I immediately contacted Personnel Department and talked back with Ms. Carol. She informed me that the hospital would do the test for latex. Finally, she gave me contact number for the Workmen's Compensation office. I contacted Ms. Cathy she took an IN-TAKE interview over the phone. When I met with Ms. Cathy in the office, I signed the IN-TAKE interview. Before leaving the office, she asks me did I contact Workmen's Compensation office before. I told her yes I did and I talked to Ms. Tammy, she informed me that this office could not help me. Despite I had allergic reactions after I did two Chemotherapy IVs (10-23), and my Supervisor sent me to ER. I had rash on my back, shoulders, and neck, and I was in ER for two-half hours. She still said it was nothing she could do to help my situation. What was I suppose to do? Ms. Cathy said I very sorry that you did not get the help sooner, Ms Tammy was new in the office. She also said that you should have been off work. Ms. Cathy arranged an appointment with Dermatology in another hospital, for latex testing. The examination was on 11-19; Dr. Apple performed a scratch test. First he scratch my hands and then put latex gloves on my hands, and wait to see if I would have a reaction (these were no the actual glove I used at work), this test was negative. We performed another test with latex gloves this also was negative. However, she did complain that her upper arms itched during the test. Given the prolonged duration of the rash, the history was also compatible with a delayed type allergy and acute one to latex. Then latex RAST test was given, also negative. Performed IGE level was normal. Next on 12-2, the allergy patch test sees if she had any delayed type hypersensitivity and this was performed on 12-5 and 12-7 reading were most important was a popular eruption to PPDA which is a component of black rubber. In addition to these reactions, he had new reactions and most significant being a significant popular reaction to the rubber chemical carbamate also known as Carbomix. This component not only has carbarmates but also a rubber chemical call DPG. The Doctor stated that this aggravating of eruption on her skin initially suggestive of an acute type reaction on rubber glove into the work place. Removal from the work place with out treatment resulted in clearing of the eruption Marion Daney has work related rash. I think there is a substantive reason to believe that she has a work-related or a work-aggravated condition. Her systematized complaints are beyond the scope of my comprehensive but I believe hey certainly should be looked into, as the sequel of not investigating could be far more life threatening than a mere skin rash would be. On March 10, 1997, I received a letter to be evaluated by Phoenix Evaluation with Dr. O'Neal. Alexis Insurance Company sent me to be evaluated. His impression is that Ms. Daney is latex allergic. She should avoid working in an environment where latex is presence. She developed a generalized dermatitis after exposure to latex gloves or in the environments where she was exposed to aerosolized latex. She had a patch test December 6, 1996. Where, she was found to be allergic to black rubber and carbamix. I was sent by my job to get an X-Ray of my lungs to see if I had smoked. Since I was not a smoker of course, my lungs test come back clear. During the Month of March Human Resources told me that they were going to place me in a job. I would have to create a new resume and I did so. In April I talked to Ms. Cathy in Worker's Compensation, she stated that we do not have a job here for you. I will send you to be rehabilitated for a job. I received a notice to report to CRA rehabilitation to help me be placed into job, June 1997. During June 1997, I wrote my resume and the CRA typed the resume and helped me to leads on a job as well as set me up for interviews. During September 1997, as the weather changed I noticed that the cool air started to bother me when I inhaled it. My chest would tighten up and I would have shortness of breath. In September 1997, I cleaned my house with pine-sole later that day used an air-fresher. I noticed later I felt tightness in my chest and I took diphenhydramine, which was prescribed by the doctor. It took about a week before my reaction was gone. I noticed that my lungs became very sensitive to every chemical, especially cologne, air fresheners, fumes outside, tires, and strong odor started to bother me. When an odor was too strong, I had to cover my mouth hold my breath and get out of the areas as fast as I could. Therefore, I would not have allergic reactions. In October, I had to take a bus because my car was in the shop. On the bus, a woman told me that she worked in an Adult Care. The fumes from the bus were strong and I could smell the tires. Then a woman got on the bus with a lot of cologne on. I did not think anything of it. Later that night I felt my chest tighten and some shortness of breath. I took Benadryl and that helped some. My reaction did not clear up. I went back to the Doctor's office and I explained my condition to Dr. Greeyt. The doctor prescribed Prednisone and Benadryl I had to take it for 15 days. I still had to continue to go to the CRA rehabilitation office after I had the reaction. Nevertheless, I noticed that the medication was making me sleepy, my heartbeat was faster and racing, the medication made me nervous while I drove my car. My Attorney informed me, that the latex would make you more sensitive. I had no way to understand until these things started to happen to me. My life is turned upside down and all around and back again. I cannot go shopping, have a good time, and not forget about my latex issues. I always have to be aware of all of my surrounding at all times. Therefore, I could avoid reactions that are very hard to do. People that wear colognes, perfumes, odors exist everywhere you turn, and the air almost impossible to not encounter (wearing a scarf over my mouth), the only place I am safe is at home. When I clean, I have to use Murphy's Oil Soap and take a bath in Mild soap like Ivory, Dove, and Oil of Olay. Therefore, I will not have to go back to the hospital to be on Prednisone again. That was a very dramatic situation and I was very upset then. Because I had to have, my friends and family drive me to the store. I could not believe that all of this was going on in my life, as soon as I felt better, I could have some control. I went to another Doctor. Who was supposed to be an expert on latex? I had the prick method testing to extract of non-ammoniated control. Hemo response to the negative saline control. I had to take the RAST test, which was a blood test, later it came back negative. Even though I had a reactions itching on my back and arms during the testing processed, that was not enough for the doctor. He only had patients allergic to latex that would break out in hives and whelps right away. He was crazy, those patients that had those reactions were having Anaphylaxis Reactions. Therefore, he was not use to patients that have a delayed reaction. So if I would have rolled on the floor gasping for air and going into Anaphylaxis Shock. Only then, he would believe me. I must be half dead before he would say, oh yeah she is allergic to latex. He stated in his report that this patient could return to work without risk of severe reactions to latex, however she should be carefully observed and be in an area where adequate medical attention could be immediately available. If she were to have untoward reaction, the patient was prescribed Zyrtec 10mg once a day to try to help reduce her complaint of itching. He prescribes for me Albuteral Inhaler as a prescription. Experts? What a laugh. Even though some doctors are aware that the RASH test is only 70% to 80% accurate. This can be very dangerous situation for people especially if some one needs surgery. If they are not aware, they are allergic to latex. It is possible they could go into anaphylactic sock on the operating table. In January 6, 1998, the Insurance Company contacted me and I was told that I had to go to another doctor. The Dr. Jack office was in Dearborn, he was supposed to be an Allergist. I told him about all of my reactions. The doctor gave me the RAST Blood test and examination. When I received his report, he stated that I could return to work and with no restrictions and that, I could return to my same job. I was so upset I cried I could not imagine being in the hospital working again. Because I know that, I had at least five reactions while working in that hospital. I know the more you are exposed to latex the more severe the reactions can be. I was appalled and frightened to death. He did not think my condition was job-related. So therefore, the Insurance Company stopped my check as of February 19, 1998. Going back to work was a death trap for me. It was too much for me to entertain the thought. I could go into Anaphylaxis Shock, which my respiratory system could shut down and my heart could go into distress. I contacted my Attorney and he said that if they want you to go back to work you must. I said Ok I would, even though I was terrified. I contacted Ms. Cathy in Worker's Compensation office I explained my situation. I told her that the doctor said for me to return to work with no restrictions. Ms. Cathy said that she was not aware of the letter at this time and that her mail did not come as of yet. When the mail arrives, I will contact you Ms. Daney. On Tuesday February 24, 1998, I contacted Personnel office and the manager stated you did the right thing to contact Worker's Compensation, now you just have to wait on their response. I contacted Worker's Compensation again on February 26, 1998 I had to leave a message with Ms. Tammy for Ms. Cathy. She was occupied at the time and could not receive calls. I left my name and phone number and I stress that I was waiting to hear form her because I needed the doctor said I was to return to work. My Attorney contacted me regarding my case. He demanded my medical records and questioned them about what were they going to do about my job. As of March 12, my Attorney did not receive any information regarding my case. So therefore, he asked me what he should do. He stated that we could sue them so I agreed. Therefore, my Attorney filed papers for my Worker's Compensation case. At that time, I only had one check coming. What was I going to do? I had to swallow my pride, and go apply for assistance at Family Independence Agency. It was so humiliated! I went to the Social Service Office on February 23, 1998 to apply for help. This was for my son and me to survive. My Social Worker name was Ms. Jackowmocy, she introduced herself. She was very kind and compassionate to me. I explained to Ms. Jackowmocj my situation, and I gave her all the papers needed for my case. As I was talking to her I was trembling, crying, and I was very upset. After I finished the paper work at Social Service, she informed me that I had to apply for Social Security Office to apply for Disability. When I received my Medicaid Card, I went to the doctor to get Pulmonary Testing at Dr. Bratt's office; this was for monitoring my breathing pattern. Even when I went into a hospital, I would get shortness of breath. The doctor prescribed me two Inhalers, Flovent 110mg (two puffs twice daily), Max-air (two puffs four times daily), EpiPen Auto Injector, use only in case of Anaphylaxis reactions, and Benadryl 25mg as needed. After going to the doctor on a regularly, the doctor made me feel as though I was stupid. Dr.

Brat's said that Ms. Daney has been diagnosed with allergic rhinitis, mild intermittent asthma, and per her evaluation with Dermatology, contact dermatitis, secondary to rubber accelerators. Ms. Daney continues to complain of difficulties with burning in her chest, as well as shortness of breath. She associates these problems as being exposed to noxious smell such as perfume or being in an environment where she suspects latex to be present. Her exam today was largely unremarkable, although she states that since being in clinic that her lungs "hurt." It is my clinical impression that much of her current symptomatology seems to have a large emotional overlay on it. Once again, we have had no evidence that she has had generalized allergic reactions to latex. However in the event that this situation may have changed, we did draw another blood test. We also gave her a new inhaler to see if this may alleviate some of her symptoms. I continued to get pulmonary testing by another doctor At this time I choose to do some research on latex, so I knew some of the problems that latex allergy caused. Of course, the doctor tried to put it off that I blew everything out of perspective it was in my head I was prescribed Singular and I was told that I now have Asthma. I never had Asthma before until I worked in the environment where latex was presence. I was not a smoker or a drinker I did not do this to myself. It seemed as though time went by my breathing got worse. I decided to see another doctor in the same office, because my present doctor did not take me seriously and he said to me. Yeah you say that your lungs bother you when you come into the hospital and he threw his hand up in the air. I refused to see him any more because it seems as though he was making fun of me. I was very upset. I was not going to be responsible for my actions if I had to continue to see that doctor. I wanted to put my hands around his throat and choke him and let him know how it was to gasp for your breathe. My Pulmonary testing result were not good, I failed the test every time I took it. I realized that I had to stop going to places where loud odors, perfumes, rubber materials, cool-cold-hot air was presented at times I had not choice. However, I had too held my breath and cover my mouth to avoid reactions from the environment. I saw another doctor in the same office always the same diagnosis, treatments, and prescriptions. Dr. Elizabeth ask me how I was in doing, I told her not so well. I told her sometimes I get pains in my chest. It feels like my heart is hurting. Dr. Elizabeth explained to me that I know you are under a lot of pressure and stress and because you are. You can cause yourself to have a heart attack, are you aware of this. After she told me that, I was afraid and after that, I tried not to get so upset, and the pain stopped. I did not want to die. My Attorney sent me to be examined at BI County Clinic P.C 1998, Dr. Albert opinion following review of the history and physical examination as described above. Marion Daney, who was allergic to latex material, developed bronchospastic lung sensitivity because of recurring and prolonged exposure to latex particles in her are of work. Further, as a result of the bronchospastic pulmonary condition, she now is not only sensitized to latex particles, but other pungent fumes, odors, and particles, colognes, rubber products and chemicals – all of which can cause sudden and severe shortness of breath and chest pain. Further, the sensitization to latex also causes and /or significantly contributes to localized and /or generalized urticaria, allergic skin reaction at exposures. Therefore, in my opinion, because of the above stated condition, she is totally disabled from returning to her previous employment and any further gainful employment, which brings her into contact with general public and/or workers who use perfumes or colognes. Further, temperature changes such as hot or cold ambient temperature can likewise trigger a bronchospastic pulmonary reaction with shortness of breath and chest pain. Therefore, she would likewise be restricted form working in these environments.

My Attorney continue to work on my case, of course they denied the cause of my condition. This just put my life in a tale spin and I was indeed losing my mind. I decided to go to Therapist. I contacted Mental Health and my approval for St John Hospital. I arrived half-hour early before appointment to fill out necessary papers for my treatment. I then meet Dr Fall; he listened and immediately wanted to get me into group therapy. I was discussing my situation I was trembling and my eyes were full of tears. When he left to arrange therapy, my tears fell down my checks. When he came back in the room, he stated that I was in a state of depression. I tried to go to group therapy I signed all the papers while I was in St Joseph Mercy Hospital downtown Mount Clemens. I had to go outside to continue to fill out the papers because I started having reactions from the latex in the air of the hospital. After I completed the papers, I was denied treatment, because my insurance would not cover that particular group therapy I was relieved because the sessions would have been inside the hospital I was having reactions just being in the hallways. I could not have been able to continue therapy at this hospital anyway. I contacted Dr, Fall's office and he immediately assigned me to a therapist for treatment. She was a female and she listened and gave her diagnosis to me. She stated that I had panic disorder, deep depression, homicidal and suicide tendencies. I told the therapist that I would like to hurt my Director at my job, because she did nothing to help me. If I have died while working and what would happen to my son? Who would take care of him? What would he do without his mother? I wanted to choke the living life out of her or just blow her head off with a gun Shot her continue to shot her until I see her suffer and die. Until she would then take her last breathe, and it was over. I had no nice thoughts of her! I just wanted her to feel pain. Killing her would have gave me some relieve of being deceived because she was informed about Latex and knew that people could die. I felt as though, I was drowning in a lake and she offered me a glass of water and ask me if I was thirsty. My reasons for feeling this way were justified. Because when I worked in Pharmacy, I was required to do IVs for patients that were allergic to latex. The procedure was different, we had to put the medication through a pour hold instead of administered the medication through the part of IV bag that contained latex. I never received any written information on the procedures or on latex allergies. Therefore, during my research I found out that other hospitals all over the country were having the same problems dealing with latex allergies. This was a big concern because doctors, nurses and other medical staff were even having anaphylaxis reactions, going into anaphylaxis shock and some even died also this included patients The Pharmacists are required to go to seminars and they have different meeting with other hospital so I know they did receive latex allergy information. I realized that the Director chose to be ignorant, but I had to pay the ultimate price, which were my health and my well- being. If I saw her today, I did not believe I could be responsible for my actions. I have suffered a great lost and apart of who I am. I do not even know this person inside of me anymore. I was being honest with my therapist and most of all myself. I had appointment with Dr.Fall to get my prescription for my depression. I received Paxil 5mg-10mg after I received he test result from my blood work. When I started taking Paxil, it did help me to begin to be relaxed at times, helped me sleep, and helped me with my mood swings. While getting therapy I had five therapists, repeating my nightmare repeatedly. It was unbearable. None of therapist ever heard of latex allergy, trying to explain my reactions to them. They just grasp it; some of them felt it was in my head. The doctor diagnosis as followed: deep depression, panic disorder, post-dramatic stress, suicidal tendencies, trembling and shaking, and etc. I did not realize that my life was so out of control. It seems as though I was eating, drinking, dreaming, smelling talking, walking and my world was all about latex. I was so absorbed in to the latex world I knew no other world. I started to research latex and documenting things that I found and collecting articles off the library computers. I was so abscessed and lost into that world nothing else mattered to me. There have been many days that I dreaded going to therapy. Because I had to tell my story repeatedly and most of the time I would cry all the way home. Wishing I could just run my car into a ditch, or just drive and drive for ever until I could not drive any more. I even thought of driving my car on a bridge and driving straight into lake. Then I would not have to live into this latex world. I would be free! Thank my lucky stars a bridge is not around the corner. I realize that I cannot give up; something inside of me just says you cannot leave your son Motherless. What message would I send to my son that his mother would not stay here and fight? She just gave up. Giving up would be too easy for me. Where is my faith? Where are my Dreams? What about fulfilling my Destiny? What about embracing Love that is all around me? I prayed to my Heavenly Father and I had questions for him. Why did this happen to me? What do I suppose to do about this situation in my life? I pray for love to be with me always and I pray for Wisdom, which I will need to help me listen to hear my Heavenly Father's voice when he speaks to me. No matter what he tells me to do, I will follow his voice. I know that he will lead me to victory. I know that my Heavenly Father gave me the gift of writing. My poetry that I write is full of love, hope, and wisdom, my poems is a reflection of my Heavenly Father's love. I realize that I can make a different and I can help others that are dealing with the same situation that I am going through. Most of all providing people with vital information on latex allergy, so that they can avoid unnecessary exposure to latex if they are allergic. Meanwhile my Attorney Mr. Berlin continues to work on my Worker's Compensation case. After a couple of postponements, finally I went to court on November 3, 1999. While the hearing in courtroom was going on, I had difficulties with my breathing. The airs from the vent in the courtroom were giving me big problems. The Employer's Attorney spoke first, and then my attorney Mr. Berlin spoke on my behalf. Then the Judge asks me to approach the witness stand. As I began to speak, the judge interrupted and made a statement. He said you are having difficult speaking. I said yes I am judge. As I finished my statement, my employer's attorney made comments. The Attorney stated that she is making this breathing problem on my own. I continued to tell the Judge about my case. On May 1994, I was hired as a Pharmacy Technician at the hospital in Pharmacy Department. When I began my training, I was to work on the baby doses and other duties assigned by the Pharmacist. In September 1994, I began training in the IV room. I learned dosing for Chemotherapy IVs; I was required to use latex gloves. I noticed that I was started breaking out on my hands. I reported the incident to my Supervisor and Management; nothing was ever done to help my situation. I continued to work in Pharmacy I decided to use vinyl gloves under the latex gloves in hopes that it would resolve the problem that I was having with the latex gloves. I thought my problem was over. I continued to have a runny nose and sometimes I became nauseas. When I was assigned to work in OR Pharmacy for five days, I noticed that that on the fifth day. I started to itch on my legs at 9 am I took my lunch at 12am – 1pm, when I came back to Pharmacy the itching started again but it got worse. The itching progressed to my upper arms and my back. I reported the incident to Gary the Pharmacist on duty. Gary said to me that Marion there is nothing up here in OR but latex, you must be allergic to latex. I reported the incident to my Supervisor, and nothing was ever done for me. Then I told the Judge about the allergic reaction that made me go to ER for two-half hours. All of a sudden, the Judge interrupted me and said stop. The Judge recalled a recent case in his courtroom. There was a young woman working in the hospital in the janitorial department. She was having allergic reactions to the latex gloves she was using. The hospital changed the young woman's position and gave her a job as a clerk in the lobby. She continues to have allergic reactions to latex, even though she did not use the gloves any more. The Judge said that I am aware that latex is everywhere in the hospital. The Judge looked at me and stopped the employer's Attorney from saying anything and he told me to leave the courtroom immediately. My Attorney approached me after leaving the courtroom, and he made a statement," You did well in court." My Attorney also told me that the court would send you the decision after the holiday. Within two weeks I received a noticed that the company wanted to settle the case. I agreed to accept the offer from the employer in February 1999. I continued with therapy because I still was having problems with sleeping, eating out of control, panic disorder, deep depression, suicidal impulses, fears of cracking up or going crazy, fears of heart-attacks and dying, trembling or shaking, and etc. I ended up with four different therapists this was beyond my control. Sometime I would break down in the office. I just could not help it. I would cry all the way home while driving the car. Trying to put my feeling in perspective. I felt as though I was dead inside, dying inside wondering if this nightmare would end. I was continuing to fill out papers for disability. The doctors did not understand my condition and they did not seem to have any patience with me, so I switched to doctors in the Macomb area. I said a pray, please let someone understand something about latex allergy. Therefore, I went to another Dermatologist hoping he can help me. Dr. Bow listened to my nightmare and I gave him a copy of my medical records. He had no clue, he did not know that the patch test had components of rubber and he gives the test to his patients. He said well you know more about this that I do. Therefore, this was a complete waste of my time again. He referred me to an Allergist. I proceeded to go to Dr. Will the Allergists, I told him about my latex allergy. I told him that I needed to be tested again for my medical records. At first, he was hesitated and wanted to test me for everything else. Finally, he gave me the Patch Test I requested. This test had the components of rubber plus other elements. He put the patch on my back and taped it. I had to wear the patch for 3 days and come back to the office so he could read the results.

He was putting me in. He looked at my back and could not see any break outs, he did not know what to do. He gave me cream that would stop the itching. A nurse came in the room and she could not understand how my back could itch just from a scratch on my hand. I told her it passed through my blood stream to my back that is what happened to me at work. She went out the room with disbelief on her face, I could not believe it. Because if something gets into your blood stream it can travel through your body. I was very angry and frustrated because I wasted my time once again. Nobody seems to understand latex allergy I was giving up. I wanted this nightmare to end! My heart went out to other people that were experience dead ends just like me. I felt so hopeless. Hell was all around me it was as if the earth was going to open up and pour out more pain. How do I continue? I periodically went to the library to look up articles on latex allergy. Once I entered the library, I had problems, because I could smell the ink and it would bother my breathing. Just smelling the in would make me sick to my stomach. I found out later in articles that ink consist of the material called latex. Now I knew why my mother's hands would began to itch when she would read the newspaper, because she had direct contact with the ink on the newspaper. My mother had to have surgery and she knew I was allergic to latex, so before surgery, she took the RAST BLOOD TEST and it came back positive. She was glad because she now had a piece of mind before she had surgery. I found one book on latex allergy in the library the name of the book was Medicines Deadly Dust A Surgeon Wake Up Call, by Dr. Richard Edlich, the book consisted of information on latex allergy and documented stories of people with the history of latex reactions. He even explained about delayed reactions to latex, which could be very dangerous. I was desperate that I wrote the doctor and I sent it to the Editor of the book, which was Vandamere Press in Arlington, Virginia. The Editor forwarded my letter to Dr.Richard Edlich who wrote the book. Within one week's time the Doctor responded to my letter. Since my phone was disconnected, I put my Mother's phone number in the letter. Dr. Richard Edlich took time out to call me and he spoke to my mother. He said that I know that she has had a rough time with the latex allergy and for me to get in touch with Latex News in Connecticut. At this time Latex News had wrote booklets on latex allergies. He wanted me to be strong and do not give up. There are people out there that understand latex allergies. I just have not had an opportunity to meet someone that was knowledgeable on the subject of latex allergy. I was overwhelmed that this Doctor Richard Edlich took the time out to call me, because he knew that latex allergy was running rapid It turned into a epidemic and the medical field and the government had to make some decisions to resolve some of the problems that latex allergy was creating. I was so touched by his call I cried, finally someone understands my pain and hear my frustrations. Richard Edlich, M.D., Ph.D., is a world-renowned authority on surgical wound healing and infection. He is a Distinguished Professor of Plastic Surgery and Biomedical Engineering at the University of Virginia School of Medicine. His gastric lavage kit for cleansing the stomach is used throughout the world. Dr. Edlich is the recipient of the highest academic honor at the University of Virginia—the Thomas Jefferson Award. There was finally light at the end of the tunnel. I contacted a hospital that was doing testing on latex patients, this was out of state. I wanted to see if I could possibility be included in the testing process. I could not participate in the testing process because the FDA had put regulations on testing in that state. The doctor told me that the RAST Test is only 70%- 80% accurate. I appreciated the doctor taking time out to talk to me and I thanked him. I wrote a letter to a Dr. Donald H. Beezghold, Ph. D who is a Scientist; he wrote an article explaining why latex testing is not accurate. The company was Latex News, in Connecticut. I wanted some help to direct me for accurate testing if possible I was desperate for answers. I wanted to know if he knew any doctors in my area that could help me with my latex allergy. I never received any response. I even wrote to JC Penny and Mervyn's asking then to donate clothing for my son. I wanted someone to hear my cry and listen to my pain. Please someone hear my Voice. I decided to go to another doctor. The clinic was a part of the University of Michigan and it was located in Livonia, in 1999. When I met my new Doctor, Dr Eileen Reichert she was very patient with me. I told her about my Nightmare dealing with being allergic to latex. While telling her my story I was trembling and she noticed that I was very upset. She took my blood pressure and she wanted me to relax. That was hard for me to do I told her. She was short and petite woman and with a soft voice, she said that University of Michigan is knowledgeable about latex allergy. I will refer you to the best Allergist that we have, Dr. Hurwitz. When she told me that I thought I was dreaming. This could not be. Yes, we can help you with the latex allergy Dr. Reichert said. Dr. Reichert impressions are as follows: She presently today in flowing approximately 30 days from now she will be evaluated by DSI for disability. Current medications include Maxair as needed, Flovent 2 puffs b.i. d. Paxil 5mg a day, Nasacort 2 sprays to each nostril q.h. s., Claritin 10mg a day, and Rhinocort as needed. She states that Paxil is not helping her with her anxiety symptoms. Whenever she takes more than 5mg, she is drowsy and cannot stay awake for the rest of the day. Friday or Saturday she will begin a small dose of Wellbutrin, at 75mg a day. She is still concern about exposure to perfumes, smells, and other types of allergens. She rides her exercise bike in her home sometimes. I hated to repeat my story but I had no choice. I made appointment to see Dr. Hurwitz the Allergist within two weeks. My mother decided to go with me because it was a long drive. When I met the doctor in the patient's room, I preceded to tell him about my Nightmare dealing with latex allergy. Dr Hurwitz said to me "Why are you upset?" I explained I worked hard to go back to school to learn a new career. I studied I worked hard to make my life better and I wanted to provide all of my son's needs. My career was taken away from me. How would you feel if you could not practice medicine again? You would not be able to help patients anymore. Your career taken away from you. How would you feel? He looked at me with a blank face. He stated that his impressions were that I was allergic to latex. I asked him was I going to be tested. He said no, because when you went to ER you had a reaction, a rash located on your back, arms, and chest it was hives. That is how latex reactions can happen. Dr. Hurwitz stated that he would write me a letter and give his impressions, I will send it to you within 10 days. I was relieved, finally someone really understands latex allergy. This doctor was my last and only hope. If he did not understand latex, I would have gone crazy. I would have committed myself; I just would not be able to handle it anymore. The doctor would have to carry me off in a straight jacket and lock me in a room. Dr. Hurwitz evaluation stated that; My impression is that the patient probably has contact dermatitis sensitivity to latex or some component of processed latex. Additionally, there may be asthma present there is definitely a good history for hayfever and the patient has positive skin tests to a number of aeroallergens. I think breathlessness and most of the respiratory difficulties are due to probably a combination on hyperventilation and vocal cord dysfunction syndrome. The patient is obviously creating some stridor. I think that some of the emotional factors-depression and anxiety disorder are contributory to respiratory status. The patient also complained of hoarse voice and difficulty breathing in a getting air in to chest. We suggested a referral to Norman Hogikyan, M.D. at University of Michigan Otolaryngology Voice Clinic in Livonia with perhaps a visit to Marc Haxler, who is a speech pathologist and could perhaps instruct the patient in techniques to keep glottis open on inspiration, would be worth while. It is possible that the patient could have symptomatic relief (respiratory), without really very much manipulation of emotional status if she is give some tools to cope with induce respiratory situation. Ms. Daney fits the profile of an individual who is likely to suffer from paradoxical vocal cord closure. The inspiratory gasping and noise that is produced sounds very much like vocal cord dysfunction. A good otolaryngology examination needs to be done to make sure thee is no vocal cord paralysis or some glottic lesion that is present, but I think that is unlikely. Dr. Norman Hogikyan, M. C. at University of Michigan performed the Laryngoscopy, flexible fiberoptic, diagnosis on April 1, 2000. I was grateful that the test I had no damage or some glottic lesions that was present. It did show that I had difficulty breathing. I had several sessions with Marc Haxler for speech therapy. Mr. Haxler would teach me breathing exercises that included walking and talking, singing Mary had a little lamb. After Dr. Reickert received the report from Dr Hutwitz, she then filled out my Disability papers. I was denied Disability once again. I had to go to court for the years (1996-1999). I had the proceeding from the Worker's Compensation case. The Dr. Hurwitz wrote in my medical file about my condition. The Judge seemed to over look some important medical information; I realized that when I received my papers from the courts denied Disability. I could not understand why I was denied I had difficulty speaking in the court, because I had a reaction and I became sick. I had difficulty breathing and talking. The appointed doctor for the disability court stated that I was disabled. She would not be able to work because of her medical condition. The Judge did not consider the doctor's evaluation. I had to appeal the Judge's decision. I had to reapply for Disability; finally, I was awarded my Disability in 2000. I continued to go to Dr. Hurwitz of University of Michigan, until my insurance changed and it forced me to go to doctors in Macomb County. I also had to change from Eastwood clinic for Psychological therapy to Oakland Psychological Clinic. P.C., I had to see another doctor. I had to repeat my nightmare again, crying and shaking telling my story. Dr. Diane had no knowledge of latex allergy. Sometimes when I explained my reactions, it seems as though people did not believe me. Sometimes it seems I was talking to the wall. The doctor reported in a letter stating my condition they are as followed: Ms. Daney was seen in the office April 25, 2001. She stated her suffering from depression and anxiety/panic disorder due to a latex allergy. She stated this allergy was preventing her from working and she was receiving disability benefits for the last several years due to the allergy and resulting depression. She has been receiving bi-weekly psychotherapy since the above –mentioned date for this depression/anxiety, ongoing latex allergy, and respiratory problems. She stated this allergy cases her much grief and frustration and prevents her from living a normal life. She states that she feels like a prisoner in her own home. This allergy has prevented her from regular motherly duties for her child outside of the home and she experiences anger and guilt. She is also having difficulty sleeping with occasional crying spells. She received treatment for the depression since 1998. My Medical doctor was Dr. Michael he was not knowledgeable about latex allergy. He referred me to a Dermatologist, Dr Sally. When I meet with Dr. Sally, I told her about my medical condition. I ask her do she do patch testing, she said yes I do. I told her that the patch test has components of rubber; this test will prove I am allergic to latex. Dr. Sally told me that she was not aware that the patch test had components of rubber, she also said well you know more about it than I do. She then referred me to an Allergist.

When I came back to the office, I had different doctor. Dr. Apple took the patch off my back. I told her I was a Pharmacy Technician I have had allergic reactions to latex gloves while working in the hospital. She looked at my records and noticed that I had seen one of her Colleague's from another office. Then she said well I do not see any reactions from the patch test, so therefore it is negative. Since, you have been to my Colleague, Dr. Lame for testing for latex allergy. He stated in his finding that he did not feel as though you were not allergic to latex and that is good enough for me. I could not believe that she did not even think twice about it. She took his word and never thought that it was possible that he missed something or did not understand completely how latex allergy happens. I was so upset I thought to myself that B_____. She did not even take the time to listen to me, where was her compassion or her patience. I took the scratch test again, that is when the doctor scratch your hand and then put the latex glove on and wait to see if there is a reaction. While the testing was going on after a couple of minutes, I noticed that my upper arms and back was itching. I informed the doctor immediately, because he did not see whelps or rash he felt as though the test was negative. Then, Dr. Will admitted to me that he never had a patient with latex allergy. So he did not even have a clue to the danger that he was putting me in. He looked at my back and could not see any break outs, he did not know what to do. He gave me cream that would stop the itching. A nurse came in the room and she could not understand how my back could itch just from a scratch on my hand. I told her it passed through my blood stream to my back that is what happened to me at work. She when out the room with disbelief on her face, I could not believe it. Because if something gets into your blood stream it can travel through you body. I was very angry and frustrated because I wasted my time once again. Nobody seems to understand latex allergy I was giving up. I wanted this nightmare to end! My heart went out to other people that were experience dead ends just like me. I felt so hopeless. Hell was all around me it was as if the earth was going to open up and pour out more pain. How do I continue? I periodically went to the library to look up articles on latex allergy. Once I entered the library, I had problems, because I could smell the ink and it would bother my breathing. Just smelling the in would make me sick to my stomach. I found out later in articles that ink consist of the material called latex. Now I knew why my mother's hands would began to itch when she would read the newspaper, because she had direct contact with the ink on the newspaper. My mother had to have surgery and she knew I was allergic to latex, so before surgery, she took the RAST BLOOD TEST and it came back positive. She was glad because she now had a piece of before she would go and have surgery. I new doctor office was Family First; they are affiliated with Mount Clements Hospital in Macomb County.

Dr. O'Connell was my doctor and I told him about my medical history. August 21, 2001. Repeating my Nightmare once again. He knew very little about latex allergy I was not surprised. He was very kind and understanding, these are his finding, I first saw Ms. Daney August 7, 2001. She has past medical history, which includes asthma, latex allergy, vocal cord dysfunction, anxiety and depression. I had to change to the Community Mental Health Services. Because Oakland Psychological Clinic, P.C. did not take my new insurance plan. Since I appealed the Judge's decision denying back pay for 1996-1999, I received a letter from the Appeal Board giving approval, and I was given a court date, September 2002. I also received papers to go to be evaluated by Social Security doctors. One of the doctor office I went to I was getting sick from the scents in the air. The doctor asks me how I was doing. I told her that my lungs were sensitive to the smell in the office. She made me take a test, put blocks in certain order, and showed me pictures and ask me what I made of the pictures. I was shaking, crying, and confused of some of the questions asked. I was angry and upset going through this process again and I told her that. I did not know why I had to come again. The next doctor I was to be evaluated by was the Psychiatrist, my sister took me to the office. There were two people in the office, they stated asking me the questions all over again. I was trembling and crying, I could not help it. Talking to the doctors became more difficult for me. All of a sudden, my voice became hoarse, and I could not speech up. I told them that I had Vocal cord problems. I feel they thought I was faking. However, I was not, my voice just became hoarse. I went to court with my Attorney. The case was discussed which including all medical records. For some reason I was denied back pay, and in the processed some how my disability was resolved. My Attorney realized it was a mistake and he revolved the mistaken and I did receive my Disability again. While waiting for the papers in the mail. I had to sign up for Disability again, I was so upset after filling out the papers. I walked in the middle of the street not even realizing the light was green. I called my therapist right away and I explained I need to talk to someone immediately. She stated I could not see you now. I told her anyone! I need to talk to someone. I was on the verge to lose my mind. I had to call another office, and they gave me emergency help line. Later that day my therapist called me back and made time for me. I realize now that if a person were on the verge of suicide they would do it because someone did not take time to listen or give them a phone number so they could just talk to someone. While at Community Mental Health Service, I was to be evaluated: Dr. Bird is seeing Marion every four weeks. Medication Review period took place on 6-30-03 on 7-28-03, 09-08-03. During the review period, Marion has experience side effects of her medications including involuntary tongue movements and her left eye not opening in the morning which she attributed to Zyprexa, just prior to the service review period. Medications have been changed in this reporting period. Her medications include Zoloft 100mg-1 and ½ pills q hs, and Vitamin E 400 mg BID. Marion reports in the past she had more paranoia, which she felt people were watching her all the time. She lost a couple of pounds, her eyes have been bothering her, and she says she cannot exercise. Ms Daney reports that she is trying to eat better 9-17-03. At this office, I had four therapists.

I had to be evaluated by a new Allergist, Dr. Hughes April 18, 2002. He was aware of latex allergy, and he had some knowledge. This is a brief follow-up letter concerning your patient, Marion Daney. She had previously been fully evaluated by my associate, Dr Andrew Staricco. His findings are the same and I will recapitulate them a bit later in the body of the letter. Marion comes in today complaining of her usual symptoms which including difficulty breathing. She has multiple things that trigger her breathing disorder, including cold air, warm air, perfumes, dust, etc. She has been seen and evaluated by multiple other physicians and also has a history of a Latex Allergy and has been disabled according to her underlying conditions.
IMPRESSION: 1. history, 2. Vocal cord dysfunction 3. History of asthma with multiple triggers, as outlined.
RECOMMENDATIONS: 1. patient continue her present regimen
2. She should continue Flovent 110 mcg two puffs twice daily and Maxair inhaler as needed. She should avoid known triggers as to not exacerbate her underlying asthma 4. Repeat her pulmonary function tests

I still go to Family First today, the doctors I have seen are Dr. Loren DeCarlo. D. O., Dr. Kristin Beougher, D.O. My doctor at this time is Dr. Kelly Bannow and now she is married and she is Dr Kelly Purcell. I still have the same medical problems and my doctor prescribed these medications: Atenolol 50mg, Hydrochlorothiazide 50mg, Lisinopril 10mg, Diphenhydramine 50mg, EpiPen Epinephrine Auto- injector for Allergic Emergencies (Anaphylaxis)

My Allergist is still Dr. Hughes, which his office is part of St John Heath Systems. The medications that Dr. Hughes prescribed are Advair Diskus

100/50, Maxair, Allegro-D., and Flonase. I still have the same Respiratory problems things have not changed.

At the end of 2004, I no longer was treated for depression at The Community Health Systems. I have a new Psychiatrist and his name is Dr. Robert Piccinini. D.O. I was frustrated because I had to tell my story once again, the nightmare that I had to face every day of my life. Dr. Piccinini asks me how Zoloft was working out for me. I told the Doctor that I still had problems sleeping and the medication made me have loose bowel, I did not like the side effects of the drug. Dr. Piccinini was very kind and patient with me, then he suggested that he could change my medication. I said whatever. The Doctor prescribed Lexapro 10mg, he said there are side effects. If you have, any problems with Lexapro contact me. I was given samples, until my next appointment. I did not have any problems taking Lexapro, so when I returned to Dr. Piccinini he continued with the same medication for my treatment for depression.

Marion Ronee Daney

DEPRESSION IS IT FANTASY OR REAL?

If you were to ask me what was depression years ago? I would not be able to answer the question. If you were to ask me now, I would have an answer. Wow, so much has happen to me I have to try to remember. When I went to Psychiatric office, I was in tears just thinking of the nightmare that interrupted my life and decided to stay to taunt me. I could not even bare talking about it, because it seems as though my heart was ribbed right out of my chest. I feel that I was walking into another world. This world took my soul, heart, and my breathe of life. I did not even know if I could get them back. The doctor prescribed Paxil 10mg; this medicine was to be taken one time daily at bedtime. The doctor wanted me to start taking therapy sessions immediately. As I continued to tell him my nightmare, I was trembling and the tears continued to flow down my face. The medicine did help me to relax and sleep sometimes. The doctor and therapy did not understand anything about latex, which I was not surprised. Every time I had a session, I dreaded it. I cried going home after the sessions. Sometimes I wish I could drive off a bridge and then my Nightmare would end. No more Latex World for me, I would have escapes the Raft of her Torching my Soul. I continued going to office and I had five therapists. Telling the story over, over, and over for me was difficult. Reliving the pain was unbearable. I had no choice in the matter. The doctor diagnosis with deep depression, panic disorder, post-dramatic tress, etc. This below is The Burn Depression Check list:

Place a check (x) in the box to the right category to indicate how much this type of feeling has bothered you in the past severally days. (0 not at all) (1 somewhat) (2Moderately) (3 a lot)

Noted by Therapist (Extreme Anxiety, Panic Attacks 04/26/00

THE BURNS DEPRSSION CHECKLIST*

1. Sadness   3
2. Discourage   3
3. Low self-esteem   3
4. Inferiority   3
5. Guilt   3
6. Indecisiveness   3
7. Irritability   3
8. Loss of Interest in life   3
9. Loss of motivation   3
10. Poor Self-image   3
11. Appetite changes   3
12. Sleep changes   3
13. Loss of sex drive   3
14. Concerns about health   3
15. Suicidal impulses   3

THE BURNS ANIXIETY INVENTORY

1. Anxiety, nervousness, worries, or fear	3
2. Feeling that thing surround you are strange or unreal	2
3. Feeling detached from all or part of your body	3
4. Sudden unexpected panic spells	3
5. Apprehension or a sense of impending doom	3
6. Feeling tense, stressed, "stressed, ' uptight,' or the edge	3

Anxious Thoughts

7. Difficulty concentrating	3
8. Racing thoughts	2
9. Frightening fantasies or daydreams	3
10. Feeling that you're on the verge of losing control	3
11. Fears of cracking up or going crazy	3
12. Fears of fainting or passing out	3
13. Fears of physical illnesses or heart attacks or dying	3
14. Concerns about looking foolish or inadequate	3
15. Fears of being alone, isolated, or abandoned	3
16. Fears of criticism or disapproval	3
17. Fears that something terrible is about to happen	3

Physical Symptoms

18. Skipping, racing, or pounding of the heart (palpitations)	3
19. Pain, pressure, or tightness in the chest	3
20. Tingling or numbness in toes or fingers	2
21. Butterflies or discomfort in the stomach	2
22. Constipation or diarrhea	0
23. Restlessness or jumpiness	3
24. Tight, tense muscles	2
25. Sweating not brought on by heat	2
26. A lump in the throat	1
27. Trembling or shaking	3
28. Rubbery or "jelly" legs	0
29. Feeling dizzy, lightheaded, or off balance	2
30. Choking or smothering sensations or difficulty breathing	2
31. Headache or pains in the neck or back	2
32. Hot flashes or cold chills	1
33. Feeling tired, weak, or easily exhausted	3

DEPRESSION
THE MONSTER

When is the rage going to stop! Sometimes when I think of my life, the rage overcomes me. How will I make it go away? Writing the book about latex will take some of my pain away. Giving all of my words, and writing down so that my voice can be heard. I realized that there are many people affected by the monster that decided to stop into my life. The Monster gave me so many Nightmares that at times I wanted to destroy my own life and I wanted to just disappear. Thank Yahweh for the Gracious of the Heavens opened up to save me. The Universe opened up her arms and gave me the Love and the Strength to continue. So many people have suffered the same anguish that I have. Tucking it away does nothing. Anger will speak and make her mark. The cries are chilling and I can hear the voices calling and reaching out for Mercy and Hope. Someone has to make a stand for all the weak and bruised Spirits. So then, I can know that they did not stand alone in the Cold, Empty Darkness. The light is there and their Voice, will be heard. This is my Destiny!

These are Letters that I wrote because I was so Desperate for someone to ear my cry

August 26, 1999 Mervyn's Corporation
22301 Foothill Blvd.
Haywood, CA 94541

Marion Ronee Daney

J. C. Penny
P.O Box 10001
Mail Stop 7303
Dallas, Texas 75301

Dear Customer Service Manager,

Hello, how are you doing today? Find I hope that the sun is always shinning in your hearts and minds. Hello, my name is Marion R. Daney, I shop at your store for my son Jonathan D. Daney. When I have the extra chance, I do. I really like your clothing for my son. I buy him Levi or the Jeans, shirts, etc., the clothing is very curable and washes very we. I have pants that are three years old and the seams are still together. I am pleased with the clothing so much that I must put it in writing so you know that I am the customer that is happy. I so have a charge but at this time, I can only pay for on it, which I was happy I could keep it. It saved me last year because I was able to charge booths for my son and me. Therefore, at this time in my life I cannot afford to buy my son any clothing. I was working at a hospital everything was on track in my life…Until I found out that I was allergic to latex. It was hard for me that I had to go to ER while at work. As I continued to work, I had other problems that accumulated. Which I was unaware that happened at the some time of being exposed to latex particles that flow in the air systems. As time went by they took me off work now I allergic to latex. They paid me for a while and then stopped paying for me. Which now I am getting Social Service, which is my only income to survive, until my job decide to start paying me again? Since being exposed to latex. I have respiratory problems. I have to use Steroids Flovent: Inhaler, Max-Air Inhaler and Singular pills everyday. The air-outside, perfumes, cleaners, tire, air conditioners, and air trigger and any strong odors now give me shortness of breath. I cannot work because now I have difficulty going places to avoid odor contact. Sometimes my reactions last 3-5 days. I do go to the doctor and he is trying to help my problems. Since latex is new they are doing the best that they can do to help me. Until then I am doomed. I am writing to you because I wonder do you donate clothing. Which my son, Jonathan need clothing for school, he is going to Clintondale Middle School, he is the Eighth Grade. I know that this is something I choose to do to write you. I had to swallow my pride. I rather eat spiders and swallow nails to make my son happy and smiling. This situation has been difficult for him. He is only 12 years old and he does not understand many things, but he is trying too. He wants things and clothing like every child would. I could not even fix his bike to ride to school or for the summer because I did not have the money. His birthday is on September 20, and he will be 13 years old I wish I could take him to Disney World but that is impossible. My wish for his birthday is that he can have enough clothes for the school Year. I want him to be like every other child and deserves better than that. My son Jonathan is caring child. All this summer he took care of an Elderly Gentleman, Mr. Fred Fischer He has Asthma and he is on a breathing machine wherever he goes. My son, Jonathan goes with him to the doctor, helps him shop in the grocery store, cooks for him breakfast, lunch, helps clean up his apartment, and most of all he always walk Hidey at lease 5 times a day. He is a good man he is well intentioned. He wants to be a Doctor or Drive Cars for designing purpose. It took a lot of strength for me to write you and I could not even hold back my tears while typing this letter. Please fine it in your hearts to help my son. I am not doing this for me. I am doing this for the love of my son. I just want him to be happy. Since my situation is like this, I cannot even have a phone.

Thank you very much for listening to my words of tears, I also like to than you for taking the time to care.

Sincerely Yours

Marion R. Daney

Both JC Penny and Mervyns's did response to the letter. Thank you for your recent letter requesting a discount or contributions. Unfortunately, our contribution policy does not allow direct contributions to individual or for the benefit of individuals, no matter how worthy the cause. We do make charity contributions to non=profit organizations in communities where we do business, because we believe they can best determine the proper use of the funds.

Despite our inability to assist, we wish you every success in the future. These are letters of my Desperations

June 26, 1999

Latex Allergy Newspapers
Dr. Donald H. Beezhold, Ph.D.
176 Risevekt Avenue
Torrington, CT 06790

Hello Dr. Donald H. Beezghold, Ph. D.,

How are you doing today? My name is Marion; I have read the Latex Allergy News article 1997 issue. I am glad that someone like you took time to help those who are allergic to latex. I am allergic to latex and some of the doctors than I went to think it is not proven. Even though they know that the blood test is not 100% guaranteed they want to stat that I have season allergies. Which is not true. I so have Hay fever. I am a Pharmacy Technician; I was working in a hospital. My nose would run all year around I did not think much of that. Until I was working in OR Pharmacy for five days and then my nose would run a lot and the fifth day I started itching all over my body. Then the next 10 days I did 2 IV in the Pharmacy are Chemotherapy at 10:00am to 10:30am. At 11am my back started itching and red, rash it was horrible. I informed my Supervisor, she sent me to ER. As I continued to work I would then itch all over after being exposed in the different units in the hospital. So now I went to so call EXPERT and he states that it is only all year around allergies. Now I have two inhalers and other medications also, one inhaler is steroids and have asthma, which I never had before. I also have sensitive to smell, cologne, tire, etc... which gives me shortness of breath and very difficult to go to places. I have to cover my mouth, take a deep breath, or inhale little because if I do the odors will trigger a reactions and it lasts 4-5 days. Even the cold and hot air gives me problems. I can only give you my first name.

Please help me I am desperate for a direction to get me more proof to help prove my case. I live in Michigan in the Macomb County Are. Do you know any doctors that you could inform me of I would appreciate it? Even someone like, yourself. I know I am not crazy, they are saying it is all in my mind. However, a funny thing they have not gave me back my job. I also took the patch test which component was CarboMix, which is a component of rubber which we know is from the rubber tree, it was positive Documented also I am allergic to latex but because of the blood test is not positive. Which they know it been pointed out FDA not have 100% test for latex, in the New York Times in March 1999.

Thank you very much for taking the time to read my letter. I will look forward from hearing from you. Leave a message if you fuzzy me information etc. At my Mother- Mrs. Lydia Hicks, if possible or at American Speedy Printing Centers.

Sincerely Desperate Situation
Marion R. Daney

August 13, 1999

Vandamere Press
P. O. Press
P. O. Box 5243
Arlington Virginia 22205
Attention: Editor
Attention Dr. Richard F. Edlich, MD., Ph.D.

Marion R. Daney

Dear Editor,

My name is Marion R. Daney, I am writing you this letter so that you can forward this letter to Dr. Richard F. Edlich. Since I really do not know how to reach him. I hope that you can send a copy. I Marion Daney am allergic to latex since 1996. Some of the doctors are not informed, as they should be. Once I took, the True Patch Test and the result were positive. Later I took the test and it was negative. Which I do not know how that happened. It was 2 ½ years apart. I do not know if it has anything to do with it. Because, I am not wor5king anymore. I took the blood test four times and it came back negative. Which I am going to take it once more. The doctor said that this delicate test and it should be done one more time. In addition, she said the glove test scratch for latex. Also when said the inhalation test, which I did not ever have. To see if I would sneeze or headache, and nausea. Which I was not aware of that these reactions at all. When I had the test, the doctor scratched my hand then put the glove on my hand. I did have a reaction it was itching on my back, upper arms and my back. That was not enough for the doctor. I guessed they wanted me to drop dead first to see if I reacted. I know when I inhale it I get shortness of breathe, nausea, even if I walk into another hospital. It happened at lease four times. This has made my life a living hell. All the odors trigger me to have shortness of breath now. I hope that the inhalation test goes through fine. This is a Nightmare that, I continue to deal with everyday of my life. I get reactions everyday. Now, I have asthma not a pretty picture, which I never had before. I am having a hell of a time. I have read you book and it is so informative. I am glad someone like you took the time out to write for people so that they could understand the whole picture. This situation can affect someone in everyone's life. I tell people about latex all the time. They thought I let my imagination get the best of me, it was all in my head. I could not help myself, because I wanted to understand. The more I understood the angry I got. Because I could have dropped dead with going to work and work did not help me at the time. I just do not know what to do. One doctor stated that I could do not have inhalation latex test, he was just a medical doctor. N o one knew of this test. Since my phone is disconnected. Please feel free to contact me you can leave a message at my Mother's home and here is the number.

Sincerely,

Marion R. Daney

LATEX WHAT IS THE TRUTH?

Introduction

I am writing this pamphlet to clear up some misconception concerning latex. I know that many people are not informed about latex. This pamphlet is to give some insight on how latex affects our lives. These are some of the questions that will be cleared up concerning this issue about latex. Where does latex come from? How do the manufactures produce the gloves? Who can be effective? How does the hospital deal with this situation? How do I know if I am allergic to latex? Are there reliable testing for latex? Do doctors really know how latex can affect your life? Being exposed to latex is there a long-term effect. Can latex kill me? What precautions should be taken if I am allergic to latex? Do any particle foods have anything to do with being allergic to latex? Should employees be concerned who use latex gloves on their job or be exposed to the airborne particles? What is the powder inside the gloves? What other products that are made with latex? Who has the greatest risk to be allergic to latex?

During the last 10 years, the incidence of latex allergies in the health care professionals has increased four-fold and now affects approximately 15 percent of health care professionals nationwide.

Where does latex come from?

Latex is harvested by **sap collection** from the **rubber tree**. During this process, ammonia is added immediately to prevent bacterial contamination and clumping of the latex, and the water is removed for higher concentration. The majority of the Haven brasiliensis cultivating occurs in Thailand, Indonesia, and Malaysia. The Manufacturers of the rubber products add chemicals called accelerators, About 90 percent of the harvested rubber is used to manufacture have extrude rubber products, injection molded goods, (rubber seals, diaphragms or tires for automobiles. The remaining 10 percent of harvested rubber is used in gloves, condoms and balloons. The dipped products appear to be responsible for most of the allergic reactions to natural rubber latex.

The production of latex gloves

Coagulant dipping most often creates industrial and surgical gloves, which involves use of a salt deposited on the porcelain hand-s shaped mold (former). The porcelain formers hang from a contiguous, automated production line, passing through various chemicals. The formers then dip repeatedly into latex, after which they are heat-cured by over-drying. Straight dipping techniques, used for the production of very thin films like condoms and examination gloves involve the use of formers dipped direct into the latex compound (no salt used) The thin latex film is then oven-dried. The coagulant or straight dipped step is complete; the oven-dried gloves are passed through water tanks to remove water-soluble proteins and any excess additives. Gloves are then cured by vulcanization, a heated process in which the latex particles become cross-linked in The presence of sulfur. Some manufactures add cornstarch, which is known as medicines deadly dust, which applying it to the finished glove surface. When applied to ease removal from the porcelain former and aid surgeons in donning the gloves in the operating room. Some other manufacturers process powder-free gloves by coating their surfaces with gel or passing the gloves through a chlorine was makes the surface more slippery, and slicker so it is easier to put on The wash reduces the amount of allergy-causing proteins in the glove. Then the gloves are packaged

Who First Discovered Latex?
Health Response Ability Systems

The British are the first to discover latex in the mid-18ᵗʰ century, but it did not come into wide use until about 50 years age. It took several more decades before allergic reactions started to appear.

I Wonder Is This A New Problem or Old?

In Great Britain in 1979, there was a woman who reacted to her household rubber gloves.

This subject of the first report: of latex allergy in the medical literature. There were about 50 cases in European medical journals between 1979 and 1988. The Food and Drug Administration stared receiving reports in the fall of 1989, when patients were going into anaphylactic shock during the radiologic examinations for the lower tract disorders. These patients received a barium enema, so at first the barium was suspected. In some of the cases, the patients went into shock after the device, a latex cuffed enema tip, was inserted but before the barium was administered. The Manufacturer voluntarily recalled all those barium enemas on the market and replaced them with silicone cuffs instead of using latex – cuffed enema tips. In all, 16 people died.

Latex Allergy In Neurosurgical Practice
Division of Neurosurgery
Children's Hospital of Eastern Ontario-Canada
By Mazagri R: Ventureyra EC
Childs Nerv Syst (CNV0, 1999 AUG 15 (8) : 404-2

The possibilities of latex allergy and the implications of the potential life-threatening allergic reactions, among patients (spinal bifida). In addition, the heath-care professionals, and latex industry workers are discussed. Latex allergy is becoming increasingly widespread in medical and surgical practice. Although early reports of latex allergy date from 1927, only over the last decade has more attention been paid to this condition. There have been increasing numbers of reported cases of adverse reactions to latex. The reactions can vary in severity from mild to fatal. There is major problem with children with spinal bifida, and who need to undergo many major aggressive diagnostic and therapeutic procedures. In this review, we aim to emphasis some aspects of the current management of the surgical patients with the latex allergy.

Who has the highest risk to be allergic to latex?

These are groups to be considered at high risk to development of latex allergy,

1.) Spinal bifida patients

2.) Children with multiple operative procedures,

3.) Health care workers,

4.) Fruit allergy patients,

5.) Patients with a history of other allergies.

6.) Spinal bifida is most common type of birth defect; they are born with clefts in thin spinal column. When multiple levels of bony spinal column are involved, the saclike membrane covering the spinal cord forms an out pouching that extent through the skin. Also is usually associated with severe nerve defects that cause bowel and bladder dysfunction. These patients often experience repeated bladder and kidney infections as well as kidney failure. They require variety of surgical procedures and require surgery to close the skin over the exposed sac covering the spinal cord this can be immediately after birth. The spinal bifida patient is exposed to many different rubber latex products, and a great percentage is these children acquire latex allergy.

7.) Dr. Kelly explains the Children born with myelomeningocele, most of them undergo two surgical procedures during the first week of life, one to repair the spinal abnormality and the second to insert a shunt for hydrocephalus. These children were being sensitized to latex very early in life. Dr. Kevin J. Kelly a pediatrician and allergist at Medical College of Wisconsin. He conducted study of children in 1990. His findings were that children spinal bifida had a risk of a life-threatening allergic reaction during surgery that was 500 times greater than that of the children undergoing surgery. He estimated 40 percent to 65 percent of spinal bifida patient were allergic to rubber products. Other patient who have undergone multiple operations, are also at increased risk of development latex allergies.

Workers with ongoing latex exposures are a risk for developing latex allergy. Such workers include: physicians, nurses, aides, dentists, dental hygienists, operating room employees, laboratory technicians, hospital housekeeping personnel, law enforcement personnel, ambulance attendants, funeral-home workers, fire fighters, painters, gardeners, food service workers, housekeeping personnel, worker in the factory where latex products are manufactured or used can be also affected. All of these types of occupations may also develop latex allergy .The initial manifestation of latex allergy is an urticarial condition that develops on the hands, often after an initial contact dermatitis that may break down the

Skin barrier. In up to 50% of exposed persons, however, the condition also affects the respiratory tract. This occurs because high concentrations of powder on latex gloves become airborne and are inhaled by workers in hospitals and clinics. The result can be sere rhinocojunctivitis, asthma and anaphylaxis. Falsities have occurred. Approximately 15-17% of health care workers are now thought to be sensitized to latex, and many of them manifesting occupational asthma may have permanent respiratory sequelate that force them to leave their jobs. Anaphylaxis may occur in 5-10% of allergic persons.

Is it possible that we could understand how allergic reactions occur?

Latex absorption through the skin is postulated as the major route of sensitization I n healthcare workers. Body sweat inside latex gloves may make latex proteins soluble; the solubilzed proteins are then absorbed through the skin, sensitizing the wearer to the latex antigen. Friction, pressure, heat and perspiration are among the nonspecific factors that influence the occurrence, severity, and sites of involvement of allergic contact dermatitis, additionally, certain skin diseases predispose to increased incident of allergic contact dermatitis. Included among these are eczema, burned skin, and nonspecific irritated skin. Penetration allergen below the top layer of skin is essential for allergenic activity, breaking of the normal skin surface barrier by injury favors sensitization. Allergen absorption can occur through unbroken skin. Skin exposure occurs, allergic reaction usually limited to be on contact, but may progress to the other part of the body. Direct skin contact possible routes of latex sensitization include inhalation, ingestion, surgical procedures, and exposure during passage of tube into a vein the spine, or other boy parts. Exposure to airborne latex allergens in hospital seeking risk of sensitizing by inhaled allergens more widespread. Life-threatening allergic response anaphylaxis to latex exposure has been show too most commonly during surgery. During abdominal surgery, cesarean section, operative procedures on genital or urinary tracts. This situation skin barrier bypassed and latex allergen absorption occurred through lining of the internal organs.

- Three types allergic reactions to latex

    1- is an irritant contact dermatitis

    Type IV hypersensitivity

    Type I hypersensitivity

An 80% all case of contact dermatitis occurs foreign substance new to individual causes direct damage to skin. Chapped skin from hand washing detergents is typical example of situation capable of produce irritant contact dermatitis. Chemicals thiurams, used latex manufacture may cause irritant contact dermatitis occurs person wear latex gloves continually at work. Mild reactions 25% to 40%. While irritant reactions do not involve immune system, they may be important contributors to allergic reaction to latex

Type I hypersensitivity reaction occurred when antigen interacts with antibody. Is an immediate reaction that can occur within minutes or 1 hour to 2 hours it can be manifest as localized hives or a life-threatening reaction with involvement of entire boy (systemic reaction) Can be skin irritation, hives, initially experience swelling of face, difficulty breathing life-threatening anaphylaxis. Airborne exposure latex allergens sensitize individual severe occupational asthma with eye nose involvement, during surgery allergens route most often associated anaphylactic reactions. Hives swelling face throat thus limiting breathing Allergic contact dermatitis low can appear similar contact dermatitis; onset irritant contact dermatitis may immediate or delayed, itching both irritant allergic contact dermatitis. Development irritant contact begins mild dryness, redness, scaling. Continued exposure, cracking, crusting, scaling of skin may occurred. Physician must have understanding patients exposure substance to plan course of differentiae the two entities Type IV hypersensitivity allergic contact dermatitis based specific allergic sensitization caused principally by skin contact with offending agent contact dermatitis allergic begins immediately or may delayed. Cases symptoms allergic contact dermatitis Type I hypersensitivity symptoms separate degrees of severity - localized hives 2) generalized hives facial throat selling 3) hives with asthma, involvement of eyes nose, ears, throat, digestive tract 4) hives with airborne contaminating involvement of the eye nose with asthma often predominates, it becoming evident some people especially healthcare workers, progress evident that people especially healthcare workers progress to long term progress to long-term asthma and lung disease. Even found that some workers developed inflammation of the heart muscle of as the result of long-term immune response syndrome.

WHAT IS LATEX-FRUIT-SYNDROME, AND WHAT IS LATEX "CROSS-REACTION"?

In Sweden at the Karalinska Hospital in Stockholm. There was a Dr I.G.K Axelesson, of the Department of Thoracic Medicine, was one of the first to describe an association between latex allergy and food.

Dr. Axelsson published a report of 12-year old girl who developed an allergic reaction with a runny nose, watery eyes and itching in the throat after eating stone fruits. Subsequently she developed allergic selling of her face and throat after inflating a rubber balloon. More recent, studies have development the existence of a "latex-fruit syndrome", predominantly affecting adult women. Also these studies confirmed that certain proteins in tropical fruits are similar to those found in latex and may be responsible for latex" cross-reaction" in certain individuals. Latex allergy has now been associated with many fruit allergies include tomato, grape, pineapple, nuts, figs, passion-fruit, celery, kiwi, citrus fruits, banana, chestnut, avocado, and peach.

Atopic individuals (persons with a tendency to have multiple allergic conditions) are at increased risk for developing latex allergy. Latex allergy is also associated with allergies to certain foods especially avocado, potato, banana, tomato, chestnuts, kiwi fruit, and papaya. [Blaco et. al 1994: Beezhold et al. 1996b.]. A group of individuals who have a personal or family history of one or more following diseases: hay fever, asthma, dry skin and eczema .The incidence of atopic in the general population approaches 20 percent. In 1993, a study done and of risk factors for latex allergy, was 94 percent of atopic patients had latex allergy.

LATEX ALLERGY COVERED BY THE
AMERICANS WITH DISABILITIES ACT

**You don't have to take it any more because THERE IS A
LAW! Latex Allergy News Volume V December 1998**

I'm mad as hell and I'm not going to take it any more! These angry words
are sounded when the unnecessary use of latex products wither exposes
us to an allergic reaction or effectively bars us from employment or access
to public and private facilities. US Public Law 101-336, better known as the
Americans with Disabilities Act (ADA), protects people with serious latex
allergy. Fair, swift, and effective enforcement of this landmark civil rights
legislation is a high priority of the federal government. You have the right to
complain directly to an offending private or public party. Absent a positive,
satisfactory response, subsequent ADA-based complaints of discrimination
are subject to government enforcement leading to ADA settlements or
Consent Agreements. For example, on October 23, 1997, the Civil Rights
Division of the U>S> Department of Justice obtained an ADA settlement and
Consent Agreement from the La Petitie Academy, Inc., a large chain of child
care centers, to modify its policies and practices for emergency treatment,
medication and staff assistance for children with allergies diabetes and
mobility disabilities. IMPORTANT: It is not necessary to have an allergic
incident before you initiate an action. The ADA public accommodations
provisions permit an individual to allege discrimination based on a reasonable
belief that discrimination is about to occur. IMPORTANT: It is usually best
to seek voluntary compliance with ADA. For example YOU DON'T NEED
A LAWYER to write a letter to the manager of your McDonalds suggesting
they discontinue the use of latex balloon premiums and /or decorations since
they deny you access or put you at risk. You can also suggest the use of

alternative latex-free products such as plastic balloons and food handling gloves. Letters from you and other interested parties (with copies to corporate management) frequently achieve successful results. Otherwise, they provide a strong basis for a formal complaint to the Department of Justice in accordance with the enclosed instructions and forms (or to the other listed government agencies). The Attorney General is authorized to bring lawsuits in cases where a pattern or practice of discrimination is alleged. In these cases, the Attorney General may seek monetary damages and civil penalties. Civil penalties may be as high as $50,000 for the first violation or $100,000 for any subsequent violation.

What is the purpose of the powder inside the gloves and what is the powder?

In 1949, Dr. R.W. Postlethwait of Duke University College of Medicine, studied the visible and microscopic tissue reaction to the cornstarch and talcum power in dogs by placing this power in almost all the parts of the body in the abdominal and chest cavity and within muscles, tendons, joints, and nerves. Dr. Postlethwait demonstrated that inflammatory reactions to talcum powder were regularly reduced in all tissues studied. In addition, the modified starch powder introduced by Dr. Lehman when placed in same tissues using identical technique produced little or no reaction. Consequently, medical science conclusively established that this cornstarch was vastly superior to, and less hazardous than, talcum powder. In. 1952, cornstarch powder had replaced talcum powder in the operating rooms of 60 percent to 90 percent of the hospitals across the United States.

Since Cornstarch is called Medicine's Deadly Dust is it safe?

A wide variety of complications caused by cornstarch have been demonstrated in literally every part of the body, Cornstarch has been reported to cause inflammation (endophthalmitis) of the eye after cataract surgery and may result in permanent loss of visual acuity. In addition, cornstarch has been reported to cause thickening of the back muscles that obstructed the connecting tube between the kidney and bladder, obstructing urinary flow. After chest surgery, cornstarch has caused a severe inflammatory reaction that produces chest pain and the development of fluid collections in the chest cavity. Aspiration of the chest cavity revealed multiple cornstarch granules. After the heart valve replacement, a patient may develop a collect; it may compress the heart chambers, markedly reducing heart blood flow. Surgical drainage of the fluid collection reveals cornstarch particles. A patient had his teeth extracted and developed tumor-like nodules beneath the gums. Some patient developed swelling of their knees, ankles and hip joints. Biopsy of the joints revealed cornstarch granules. In these cases, there was evidence that cornstarch entered the joint space during diagnostic or therapeutic procedures.

There are two approaches to prevent the adverse effect of powdered surgical glove lubricants: The first removes all trace of powder lubricants from the surface of the surgical glove that contacts the patient. (This goal of power removal is formidable take when one pair glove covered by as much as 700 mg of cornstarch power) The manufacturers have prepared warning labels on each glove packet-advising physicians to wash off the powder before use in wounds because of the toxicity of cornstarch.

In London, England in the Westminster Hospital D.G. Jagelman and Harold Ellis reported that washing reduce the number of starch granules, but left significant cornstarch that appeared to aggregate as clumps on the gloves. Cornstarch would promote a delay in absorption and enhancement of the foreign body a reaction.

In 1975, in London, England S.JS.Kent of St. Thomas's Hospital described a method of removing cornstarch powder from surgical gloves. He reported that gloves scrubbed while immersed in a bowl of 1-percent cetrimide solution and rinsed with sterile water greatly reduce the amount of residual cornstarch on the surface of the gloves.

The most effective method of washing the cornstarch from the gloves involves a 1-minute cleansing with 10ml of povidone-iodine followed by a 30-second rinse under sterile water. This technique reduced the median number of cornstarch granules per mm of glove, as seen on microscopic examination from 2,720 (when to attempt to remove the powder wade) to 0 (when the povidone-iodine method was performed.) This technique is a burdensome to the clinical staff as well as time-consuming and costly. Also, it can't ensure that all power particles have been removed. Further, it can't ensure that all powder particles have been eliminated

Marion Ronee Daney

Clinical Summary

Starch Powder Contamination of Surgical Wounds
Hunt T K, Slavin J P and Goodson W H.
Archives of Surgery.pp.825-828, August 1994
Objectives

A two-part study was undertaken by the researchers to determine whether cornstarch glove powder contaminated surgical wounds (1) despite glove washing and /or (2) when only one member of the surgical team with indirect surgical site contact wore powdered gloves.

PART
Methodology

Thirty-two operations (neck, chest, abdomen, but mostly mastectomy) were performed with surgical team members wearing wither powdered or powder-free gloves (according to individual preference immediately after donning, all the powdered gloves were washed or wiped to remove the powder. An additional 10 operations were performed with the entire surgical team wearing powder-free gloves. (Biogel).

After the surgical operation, the surgical site was rinsed with Ringers Lactate solution. The solution was collection and tested for evidence or powder granules.

Results

Despite washing/wiping, starch granules were found in the irrigation solution from all 32 of the operations during which powdered gloves were worn. The number of starch particles increased as more members of the surgical team wore powdered gloves. No starch particles were found from the ten operations during which members of the surgical team exclusively wore powder-free gloves.

PART 11
Methodology

Pathology slides from 26 mastectomy patients who had been previously biopsies were examined. Powdered gloves were worn for 11 of the biopsies. Powder-free gloves were worn for 15 of the biopsies. For the latter 15 biopsies, the surgeon wore powder-free gloves. However, the nurse who set up the instrument tray wore powdered gloves.

When analyzing results, researchers, forum starch granules at the previously biopsies site of all 11 patients during which the surgeon had worn powdered gloves for the procedure. In addition in 3 of the 15-biopsy sites during which the surgeon had worn powder-free gloves, starch granules were also present. The authors noted that for these 15 procedures, the nurse setting up the instrument tray wore powdered gloves.

Summary

Cornstarch glove powder will contaminate a surgical wound even if only one member of the surgical team with indirect surgical site contact wears powdered gloves.

Regnet Medical as a service to healthcare professionals has completed this summary of a published scientific paper. A copy of the original paper may be obtained through Regent Medical by Email or direct from the publishers of the Journal in which it appeared.

How do you Diagnosis Latex Allergies

There are several tests are available, and one been approved by the FDA (Alastat Latex-Specific IgE Allergen Test Kit, Diagnostic Products Corp. Los Angeles). These texts are limited and are 10-20% positive results may be missed. More strong specific tests are available through reference laboratories. Standardized skin test extract has not yet been made commercially available. Some clinicians have attempted skin testing with a saline solution into which a latex glove has been immersed. Some try on the actually glove wet for testing. This very dangerous and have led to systemic reactions. Specialist under carefully controlled conditions should only do this.

Latex allergy should be suspected in anyone who develops certain symptoms after latex exposure including nasal, eye, or sinus irritation; hives; shortness of breath; coughing; wheezing; or unexplained shock. A physician should evaluate any exposed worker who experiences these symptoms, since further exposure could result in a serious allergic reaction. A diagnosis is made using the results of a medical history, physical examination and test.

The first step is diagnosing latex allergy is taking a complete medical history. The Food and Drug Administration (FDA) had approved blood test, which are available to detect t latex antibodies. In addition, other test are available include a standardized glove-use test or skin tests that involve scratching or pricking the skin through a drop of liquid containing latex proteins. Itching, swelling or redness at the test site shows a positive reaction. However, no FDA-approved materials are yet available to use in skin testing for latex allergy. This test should be performed only at a medical center because they are very dangerous.

Testing is also available to diagnose allergic contact dermatitis. In this FDA-approved test, a special patch containing latex additives is applied to skin and checked over several days. Itching, redness, swelling, or blistering where the patch covered the skin shows a positive reaction. Occasionally, test may fail to confirm a worker with no clinical symptoms. Therefore, a knowledgeable physician must evaluate test results. There is another Blood Test for Latex Allergy. Diagnostic Products Corporation has received approval to market its latex allergy test (AlaSTAT), the first blood test to become available for identifying individuals who are hypersensitive to latex. The test should help physicians cope with the increasing problem of latex allergy.

The Alas TAT test measures specific IgE antibodies against latex. The in vitro test is performed on a blood simple and takes about 3.5 hours. In the four-step procedure, specific IgE binds to B-allergen. The antibody-allergen complex is then bound to a biotin-coated tube. Enzyme-labeled anti-lgE antibody is added, and the resulting complex is reacted with an enzyme substrate. If the specific anti-latex lgE i.e. present in the blood sample, the substrate reaction causes the sample to become colored. AlaSTAT is intended for diagnosis of patients with suspected latex allergy. It is not intended as a screening tool. If a patient tests, positive measures can then be taken to avoid exposure to latex products. The manufacturer claims that the test has a clinical sensitivity of 91% to 100%, and that the predictive value of a negative result is 99% for a population with a 10% prevalence of latex allergy. (Snider S. FDA Electra Bull Board. March 24, 1995;T95-16. Additional information from the manufacturer.

Marion Ronee Daney

LATEX ITEMS ARE
NOW REQUIRED LABELING

FDA rules latex devices must have warning labels. (Labeling of products containing latex which may cause allergic reactions)

The FDA had received over 1,100 reports describing allergic reactions, 15 deaths related to the use of latex-containing medical products and devices between 1988 and 1992. By 1995, there were over 1,600 reports and 23 deaths caused y allergic reactions to latex. Thousands of nurses, doctors, dentists, and other health care workers jeopardize their health and sacrifice their careers because of severe latex allergy. Modern technologic advances in latex manufacturing can dramatically reduce the allergy-provoking factors in latex. Today, latex surgical gloves with low levels of latex allergens should be used exclusively in medical practice to prevent harm to patients and staff.

Are there any solutions?

They have Low-allergen gloves and alternatives for some other products are now available, and the Medical Devices Bureau, Health Protection Branch Health Canada, published Compendium of Non-Latex Gloves in July 1994. The American Academy of Allergy and Immunology recommends the following guidelines for preventing latex sensitization until a solution to the problem is found.

Pennsylvania

Latex Allergy Awareness Week

The week of October 4-10 has been designated Latex Allergy Awareness Week in Pennsylvania following Monday's passage of resolution sponsored by Senate Democratic Leader Robert J. Mellow.

"Latex allergy is very serious and potentially lethal condition that affects millions of Americans," Mellow said. "The state should make an effort to educate its citizens, particularly those whose work demands the use of latex products, about the dangers pose to those with this allergy."

The New York State Assembly has recently passed legislation requiring the state Department to Health to complete a review of the existing research regarding latex allergies. One completed, the department will then work with medical providers to develop a latex management program for complete News Release- Contact: Bob Billstone-Phone: 717-787-6481.

Marion Ronee Daney

Patients in high-risk groups should be identified.

Latex Allergy in Neurosurgical Practice
By Mazagri R: Ventureyra EC

The possibility of latex allergy and the implications of the potential life-threatening allergic reactions among patient (spinal bifida), health care professionals, and latex industry workers are discussed. Latex allergy is becoming increasingly widespread in medical and surgical practice. **Although early reports of latex allergy date from 1927**, only over the last decade is more attention been paid to this condition. This is due to an increasing number of reported cases of adverse reactions to latex, varying in severity from mild to fatal.

1. Some patients, regardless of risk group status, should be questioned about a history of latex allergy

2. All high-risk patients should be offered testing for latex allergy

3. Procedures on all patients with spina bifida should be performed in an environment free of latex (no latex gloves, latex accessories- catheters, adhesives, tourniquets, anesthesia equipment) that comes into direct contact with the patient.

4. Patients with positive history, regardless of risk group status, should performed in an environment free of latex

5. Patients identified as latex-allergic by history or testing should obtain Medic Alert bracelet and self-injectable epinephrine.

Facts About latex Allergies
Latex Allergy Fact Sheet
Latex Allergy is an Acquired Allergy
Andover Coated Products © 2000

There was a change, and that was talc, which was heavy to cornstarch, which was a light powder. The cornstarch binds with the latex proteins and carries them in the air where there can be breathed.

The Powdered latex gloves create an aeroallergen that is inhaled and can be absorbed through even the mucosa.

The American College of Allergy, Asthma and Immunology believes that 20% of the health care workers are allergic to latex. Estimates are that 18 millions Americans are allergic to latex.

There have been 28 deaths reported to the FDA-these include reports of patient given barium enemas, children, a physician, nurses an others. There are safe alternative products are available at competitive costs.

The **FDA will require mandatory labeling** of any medical device containing latex. Which comes in contact with humans as of **September1998.**

Many of the hospital are changing to non-latex exam gloves. In addition, the hospitals have banned latex balloons.

Many health care professionals have been left unable to continue in their profession. Their health problems continued and worsen, even after leaving the hospital setting.

THERE IS NO CURE. THERE IS NO DESENSITIZTION currently available for latex allergy. We can only mediate to help decrease symptoms.

AVOIDANCE IS THE ONLY INTERVENTION to latex allergy.

RAST update
IMVS Newsletter Number 46 Winter 2002
By David Gillis

Recent improvement in the RAST Test has widened its application in clinical practice and allowed the performance of RAST testing to equal that of skin testing in many instances.

The radioallergosorbent test (RAST) has been used for many years as an alternative to skin prick teting in diagnosis of allergic disease. RAST testing measures specific IGE test to a particular allergen in conjunction with corroborative clinical history indicates that it is likely to be the causative allergen. On the other hand, a positive RAST test to an allergen, by itself without clinical history does not necessarily mean the patient will react to that allergen if challenged.

Although the RAST test when first developed, was a qualitative test express as a score
1-4, recent technological improvement has lead to its evolution into a quantitative test
(expressed in allergy units of specific IgE to allergen). Because more allergen can now be attached to the solid phase, binding of antibody can now be related back to antibody to a standard curve for total IgE that improves accuracy.

Existing indications for RAST

- Prior medication (antihistamines/antidepressants) which would interfere with skin testing

- Widespread eczema precluding skin testing.

- Young children (over 2 years old).

- Dermatographism leading to false positive skin tests.

- Inability to carry to skin testing (distance, cost etc).

Role in Latex Allergy

RAST testing in a patient with suspected type 1 latex allergy is useful if positive (a 2kUA/L). However, a negative result does not exclude the possibility of latex allergy and so patients with negative RAST testing and suspected latex allergy should proceed to skin testing with inhouse or commercial latex extract.

Marion Ronee Daney

GERMANS ALLERGISTS DEVELOP BREAKTHROUGH TEST

The Week in Germany: Business and Technology
September 24, 2004

A new test developed by doctors at Berlin's Charite hospital to diagnose allergies promises to save millions in health can delivering results as accurate as a laboratory screening at a fraction of the cost.

Doctors at the hospital's Allergy Center unveiled the device call FastCheckPc, on Tuesday.

A small plastic box outfitted with a sensitive paper strip, the FastCheckPac, works something like a litmus test.

A small sample of a patient's blood, together with a special solution, is spread onto a paper strip, which then indicates signs of 12 of the most common food and inhalation allergies.

At a price of just 17 Eur ($21), the device costs about one-teeth as much as laboratory testing. With results that are 90% to 100% accurate in just 30 minutes, the FastCheckPoc saves time as well.

"This is a bedside test, which can be carried out by any practitioner, anywhere, anytime and regardless of specialist knowledge or training," said Ulrich Wahn, a member of the development team behind the new innovation.

According to figures from American Academy of Allergy, Asthma and Immunology, some 20% of Americans suffer from, are the sixth leading cause of chronic disease in the United States.

With the number allergy sufferers expected to rise, early detection is more crucial than ever, the German team said.

"Whether cat allergy, hay fever or asthma, allergies tend to start from a young age," Wahn said reporters. "Early detection problems before they develop."

The FastCheckPoc is available to physicians now.

LEAP TESTING SERVICE

The Latex ELISA for Antigenic Protein (LEAP) Testing Service is an independent testing laboratory at the Guthrie Research Institute in Sayre, Pa Directed by David Kostyal, Ph. D., and the testing service specializes in testing natural rubber latex products, such as gloves, for the assessment of latex protein levels.

Updates:

LEAP 2 ASSAY TO BE REPLACED BY ASTM D6499-03 AS OF JANUARY 2005

With the adoption of the ASTM D6499 standard we have seen a dramatic decrease in the number of requests for the LEAP assay, which was originally developed here of Guthrie. Both assays use an ELISA based technology and are specific for latex proteins. The increase in 6499-03 requests is understandable, as the ASTM D6499 assay offers some advantages over the LEAP. It is recognized standard while the LEAP is not, and has a greater level of sensitivity than the LEAP. The costs of maintaining the LEAP reagents for the assay are not feasible and we will stop performing the LEAP assay as of January 1st 2005. Anyone who requests a LEAP assay will be informed that the ASTM 6499-03 will be performed instead.

"The ASTM D6499-00 protocol has been updated and is currently designated as ASTM D6499-03. The changes to the protocol are editorial in nature (i.e. The designation of Akron Rubber Development labs as sole the repository for the D6499 reagents, has been added.) The test method itself remains the same. We are in the process of changing our certificates to read "ASTM D6499-03" to reflect this update.

The LEAP Testing Service Receives Accreditation to the International Standard
ISO/IEC 17025 by A2LA through November 30, of 2005.

The LEAP Testing Service earned accreditation by the American Association for Laboratory Accreditation (A2LA) for technical competence in the field of biological testing, certification number 1438-01. The testing service's accreditation was expanded to include three testing methods: two Lowry-based assays –**ASTM D5712-95 and -05; and** an ELISA-based assay—**ASTM D6499-03**. This accreditation guarantees that all clients will receive the highest quality testing available for all samples submitted.

LEAP Testing Service:
LEAP was established by Dr, Beezhold in 1993 following the development of the LEAP Assay at the Research Institute. It was the first laboratory in the world to commercially test latex products by ELISA Assay and to date has tested more than 28,000 samples
The LEAP Testing Service is part of the Laboratory of Immunobiology at the Guthrie Research Institute in Sayre, Pa.

Contact Information:
LEAP Testing Service
C/o Donald Guthrie Foundation for Education Research Inc.
One Guthrie Square
Sayre, Pa 18840
Phone: (507) 882-4645
Fax: (570) 882-4666 or 882-5151 Email: LTS@guthrie.org.
Latex Allergy test Discern Which Patients Need Avoidance Management:
PRESENTED AT AAAAI

Marion Ronee Daney

Microarray-based Improvement of Diagnosis for Latex Allergy. Abstract 442

By Paula Moyer

March 23,2005-San Antonio, TX—A new latex allergy test can help physicians differentiate asymptomatic, sensitized patients from those with true latex allergy who need to avoid contact with it, according to findings presented here March 20th at the 61st annual meeting of the American Academy of Allergy, Asthma, and Immunology.

"Rather than simply identifying latex sensitivity, this test will help us know which patients are at risk of serious reactions,' said principal investigation Stefan Wagner, PHD, postdoctoral fellow, department of pathophysiology, Medical University of Vienna, Vienna, Austria. "This identifies a latex-specific allergy, in contrast to asymptomatic cross-reactivity, and therefore provides us a way of stratifying risk."

With co-investigators, Dr. Wagner sought to develop a modality that would be an improvement over currently used reagents for latex allergy diagnosis. The currently techniques identify primarily the presence of immunoglobulin E (IgE) that is specific to latex and related compounds.

The researchers developed a microarray-based latex allergy diagnositic test that uses newly generated latex protein extracts, a panel of recombinant latex allergens, and horseradish peroxidase. Horseradish peroxidase is often used in allergy tests because cross-reactivity between it and other allergens is common.

They recruited 74 subjects with a compelling history of latex allergy and a positive latex skin test (group i), 44 without a history of latex hypersensitivity but, other inhalant allergies (group 2), 29 individuals with a compelling history but negative results with skin, serologic tests, or both (group3), and 62 without symptoms but positive skin test or a capture (CAP) test (group 4).

The investigators ten tested the participants' sera with the microarray-based test.

The new test was 97.3% sensitive for group 1, of whom 83.8% had a positive CAP result. Its sensitivity rtes were 85.2% for group 3 and 98.4% for group 4. The specificity of the test was 65.9% for group 2.

Most reactions to latex allergy in group 1 were observed for the most common latex allergens—Hev b6, 60.8% of Group 1 reacted, and Hev b5, to which 31.1% fo the reacted. Those two allergens are the ones that resist the process of glove manufacturing and continue to be present in extracts of medical gloves.

Conversely, in the group of asymptomatic sensitized individuals (group 4), most reactions were detectable to Hev b8, affecting 40.4% of them, and horseradish, affecting 38.7%. In the case of group 4, this finding showed that the individuals have a less specific cross-reactivity and do not need to avoid latex unless they develop symptoms, Dr. Wagner said.

"This test is more sensitive than others currently available," Dr Wagner said. Discerning the patient' IgE binding pattern allows us to know whether they are sensitive to allergens of clinical relevance, or whether they have a cross-reactivity to less relevant allergens."

The study was funded by the Austrian Science Fund grand SFB-F01802.

Diagnosis

There are three major categories of tests for confirming a diagnosis of latex allergy: skin tests, in vitro serologic tests, and provocative tests. Most of the experts feel that a skin prick test with a diluted latex antigen extract in the most sensitive and, therefore, the gold standard for detecting latex allergy. Unfortunately, while the commercial skin prick test extracts are

Marion Ronee Daney

available in Europe (Stallergenes, Antony, France) and Canada (Bencard, Toronto, Canada),. None of these test are available in the United States. As a result, clinicians sometimes use nonstardardized, office-made extracts produced from mixing glove squares with saline. The stock solution is diluted in saline to 1:1,000,000. Testing is performed by placing a drop of diluted antigen solution on the skin and gently pricking the skin with application, the wheal is measured by adding the two largest perpendicular axes and dividing the sum by two. A positive reaction is noted at 15 minutes, then increasing concentrations are subsequently tested. While anaphylactic risk during prick testing is minimized by initially using very diluted solutions, physicians should be prepared with latex-safe resuscitation equipment and epinephrine.

Serologic RAST (radioallergosorbent) tests are in vitro tests in which solid-phrase allergen is incubated with serum to induce specific antigen-antibody reactions. Radiolabeled anti-IgE antibodies are mixed with solid-phrase allergen-antibody complexes, and bound radioactivity is measured. RAST-like tests available in the United States include: AlaSTAT (Diagnostic Products Corporation, Los Angeles CA); CAP (Pharmacia, Peapack, NH); and HYTECH) Hycor Biomedical, Inc., Garden Grove, CA). Sensitivities and specificities rang from 74% - 97% and 33% - 97% respectively. Therefore, a negative RAST does not exclude latex sensitivity. Because these tests only measure serologic antibodies, which may decrease after allergen avoidance, they do not provide quantification of latex antibodies bound on tissue mast cells.

Provocative tests include use tests and inhalation challenge tests. A use test involves applying a latex glove directly to a wet hand; a vinyl glove serves as a control. First, one wet finger is exposed to a glove finger for 15 minutes. A positive test is defines as 2-5 urticarial wheals. If no reaction is observed, the entire glove is applied to a wet hand for an additional 15 minutes. If no wheals are noted, exposure can be lengthened to several days or the test can be modified so that the skin is pricked before application of gloves. Inhalation challenge tests involve measuring spirometry at 15- 30 minutes intervals, while subjects handle latex gloves. If no reaction is detected, patients are then asked to blow up latex gloves, expelling the contents slowly into their faces, vinyl gloves are used as controls. These tests are unregulated and carry a risk of anaphylaxis.

SKINmed 2(6): 359-366, 2003 © 2003 Le Jacq Communiction, Inc.
http://wwwmedscape.com/viewarticle/464479_7

PRINCIPLED BUSINESS LEADERSHIP IN MEDICINE 16

"Every innovator has the past to contend with. It is difficult to swim upstream against established opinion."Dr. Owen H.
Wangernsteen

D r David Podell, an Ophthalmologic Surgeon, was one of the first to recognize the potential applications of hydrophilic resins like hydrogel polymers for use as coatings for biomedical devices. His office was very busy and located in New York's midtown Manhattan. Dr. Podell had been bothered for years by the seemingly ubiquitous presence of tiny powder particles from his surgical gloves. These particles frequently attached themselves to his instruments and were often visible during procedures through the oculars of his operating microscope. The doctor was aware of wealth of medical literature documenting the serious hazards of talc and Cornstarch powder glove lubricants in intra-abdominal surgery. Dr. David Podell recalls in 1970's an 84-year-old patient experience a troubling clinical problem as result of the cornstarch powder coating his surgical gloves. The elderly Haitian women had only one eye because he had lost her sight in her earlier life. She had developed cataract formation in her eye. The doctor performed the appropriate surgical procedure, intracapsular cataract extractions, with success. The patient returned with a severe inflammation of her iris after two day after the surgical procedure. When the doctor examined her eye he notice that her eye looked cloudy and demonstrated a layered level of pus in the anterior chamber, like a half-filled glass of milk. He noted that the diagnosis of early endophthalmitis (inflammation) characterized by recent hypopyon formation (pus level) and anterior vitreous cellularity (cloudiness). Dr. Podell decides to treat his patient aggressively to cover both an irritant an infectious cause. Dr. Podell continued to treat this patient for months, she even lost some sight 20/50, and she continued using medicines for her eye on a daily basis. She used topical cortisteroids and antiglaucoma treatment to control the alternating bouts of inflammation and steroid-induced glaucoma. Dr. Podell was deeply concerned and contacted someone, which they were raised as brothers Howard. He was a chemical engineer and they discussed the problems with the latex gloves with cornstarch. Dr. Podell and Howard Podell started investigating how to the process in creating the new latex glove. David told Howard of his ideal to develop a surgical glove coated with a type of plastic polymer in place of the exclusively used powdered glove lubricants. Time with patients and help from many different sources and a lot of research was involved in creating this new latex glove. Dr. Podell through his dedications and concerns for his patients the glove that was manufactured was called hydrogel-coated glove gained 40 percent of the sterile surgical glove market in the United Kingdom, and they were being introduced into other European countries. He goes through a process for United States.

CAN PLAYING CHILDREN'S GAMES BE RISKY?

We all know that going to Birthday Parties is fun. All people big and small enjoy them. But you would have never thought that blowing up balloons for fun could be dangerous for some that at allergic to latex. Most people are not aware of this.

We know that baseball is loved all over the world. Softball game is similar to baseball, played with a ball called softball. There are some difference in the pitch speed, equipment, and the field size. In the United States Amateur Softball Association, with headquarters in Oklahoma City, Oklahoma, governs the sport. Softball seems to be so innocent. I wonder what is it made of? Softball is larger than the regulation baseball. It can be made of kapok (silky fiber), a mixture of cork and rubber, a polyurethane mixture, or other approved materials. The ball is hand or machine-wound with a fine quality twisted yarn and it covered with latex or rubber cement.

When Rubber Rubs the Wrong Way
By Dori Stehlin
Journal of the American Association of Nurse Anesthetists, October 1991`

Every Thursday, Sue Lockwood's eyes would start to swell. Fridays were always the worst. Sometimes her eyes were so swollen she could hardly see. But, without fail, by the time Monday rolled around, the welling was gone and her eyes were fine. "I thought that I was allergic to the sand that I was playing volleyball on every Thursday," says Lockwood, who lives in Grafton,

Wis. "The sand would get in my eyes and I thought I was breaking out from the sand". But, although Lockwood quit playing volleyball in August 1991, the problem with her eyes persisted into the fall. Two ophthalmologists told her that her symptoms didn't indicate an eye infection. Finally, in October she went to see an allergist. "After interviewing me an getting a medical history he told me he was sure I was latex sensitive. Sure enough, he drew blood and I tested positive." What were the clues that led to the allergist's conclusion? First, Lockwood is a surgical technician. Like most health-care workers today, Lockwood practically lived in latex gloves at work.

Second, her work schedule was Tuesdays, Wednesdays, and every other Thursday. That explained the miserable Fridays and recovery by Monday. Then there was the volleyball. "It turns out she didn't use a standard volleyball," says her allergist, B. Lauren Charous, M.D. "Her team used a red rubber volleyball." Few better than Lockwood the surprising places latex can show up. "I don't know what I'm going to run into next," she says. She is reacted to the new carpet in her mother's house (the carpet backing contained latex) and to her nieces' and nephews' rubber toys.

Latex Allergy from Mouthpiece
By Douglas Hoffman, MD, Ph.D.
This Village /all Health .com service

Fans can't wait until the Super Bowl in January happens. Football is another sport played all over the world. In High School the students can't wait until the season come for them to play football. To protect the players they are gear that is required. Which one on the items is a Mouthpiece? Most people would never think anything of this. But for a young man playing football putting the mouthpiece in his mouth can end up in agony. During football practice a young man had broken out in horrific sores on the sides of his mouth and has all bubbles and sores in his mouth and on his tongue. The pediatrician advised a combination of Benadryl and Maalox applied to the sores inside and out. And said to apply Neosporin to the exterior sores at night is this also called "trench mouth" or Kawasaki disease" and can something else be recommended. This is a Mother (Pat) asking Dr. Douglas Hoffman, MD, Ph. D. about her son's condition. His responses was **"Don't let him put that mouthpiece back into his Mouth!** From your description, this is neither trench mouth nor Kawasaki disease. The most likely explanation for your son's problem is latex allergy. Latex allergy is a hypersensitivity to latex or "natural rubber", a material this hasted from rubber plants. Trauma seems to facilitate development of latex allergy: if your son's mouthpiece "digs" into his oral mucosa (mucous membrane) on a rear is, he may have had ample chance to developed this hypersensitivity

CHEWING GUM CAN BE A
MOUTH FULL

I always enjoyed chewing gum. There are so many different types and flavors of gums to choose. My favorite is Bubble Gum any flavor especially strawberry. I was always puzzled why my throat would itch while I was chewing gum. The answer is in the next sentence. When I did some research on latex, I ran across an article on the Internet. At that time, I was chewing bubble gum enjoying myself. As I started to read on gum I was surprise what I found out. Gum, gelatinous substance exuded by plants. Gums are composed of complex organic acids called gum acids, or the salts of these acids. When hydrolyzed, gum acids, such as arabin, yield sugars such as arabinose, galactose, and xylose, and simple acids. Gums have a consistency similar to glue when moist but are hard when dry. They are colorless and odorless and will not dissolve in organic solvents, although they are readily soluble in water. Gums are used as a base for mucilage, in cloth finishing and calico printing, and as emulsifying or soothing constituents of medicines. Gum arabic, exudates of several species of acacia, is typical of gums that contain arabin. Gum arabic of the finest quality is obtained from Acacia Senegal and A. Arabica, found in western and northern Africa. The gum forms a clear, thick solution in water. When ethyl alcoholics added to solution of gum Arabic and water, which has been slightly, acidifies with hydrochloric acid, arabin is produced. A similar gum, cherry-tree gum is exuded form the bark of several species of Prunus, such as common cherry and plum trees. Many gum resins and other plant exudates are commonly called gums. Gum resins are substances that contain both gum and resin, so that both water and alcohol are required to dissolve them. The principal gum resins are so called gums of ammoniac, asafetida, benzoin, galbanum, gamboge, myrrh, and sandarac. Latex, from which chicle, rubber, and gutta-percha are derived, is composed of gum resins, waxes, and fats. Chewing gum is usually made form chicle.

Chicle- coagulated milky juice of the sapodilla, uses as principle ingredient of chewing gum. (Spanish from Nahuat) chictli

Resin- any of numerous clear to translucent yellow or brown solid or semisolid, viscous substances of plant origin such copal, roslin, omber used principally in lacquers varnishes, ink, adhesives, synthetic plastics, and pharmaceuticals.
21 www. Allhealth.com/conditions/allergies/qa/2,4801,41-176068,00. html

Sapodilla-An evergreen tree (Manikara Zapoto) of Mexico and Central America having Latex that yields chicle and edible fruit with sweet yellow - brown flesh, fruit of this plant also called naseberry (Spanish zapotillo, diminutive of zapote, sapodilla fruit from Nahuati tzapotl

Something Was Not Right About David!
Children Reactions
The Canadian and Americans Latex Associations
By Karen

This article goes into detail what parents can go through when a child has an allergic reaction to latex. When a couple had a child and his name was David. They something was not right. He cried a lot and seemed to have a lot of discomfort in his abdominal area. When he was one year old, they discovered he had numerous food allergies. He also had a lot of trouble with his skin. Always getting rashes and irritated by water - They spent a lot of time trying different creams. When the mother would put the cream on, he was fine. When her husband would put the cream on him, he would break out into hives all the time. The mother thought that her husband was no gentle enough. The husband occupation was a Dentist, and while at work, he would wear latex gloves. David would break out into hives, yet on the weekends or vacation he would be fine, even when her husband applied David' cream The Parent took David to an Allergist and said that they were sure that he was allergic to latex. David really did not fit the norm as children with latex allergies usually have spinal bifida. He was tested and it was positive. The parents were very upset and did not know how to turn. They even had to refuse a balloon and said he was allergic to them, but people thought they were over reacting. David was breaking out into hives from rubber boots and sometimes with new underwear. Now when the parents buy new items like underwear and bathing suits, the items are washed a few times in very hot water before he wears them

Children On Home Mechanical Ventilation At Risk For Latex Allergy
A Doctor's Guide Review of: "Latex Allergy in Children on Home Mechanical Ventilation
By David Loshak 10-23-2000

Many children who need home mechanical ventilation, while often exposes them to products made of latex, become allergy to the material. Screening might identify those with previously undiagnosed allergy and prevent reactions, according to Californian team chest physicians. While the prevalence of latex allergy in the general population no greater than 1.0 percent, it can be ash high as 60 percent of the patients with spinal bifida and other chronic medical condition associated with repeated exposure to latex. There were 57 children receiving home mechanical ventilation were given radioallergosorbent test for latex and had serum immunoglobin E (IGE) levels measured. Of the 57 patients, 17 29.8 percent) tested positive for latex. Those with latex allergy had required mechanical ventilation an average of 6.1 ± 4.1 years compared with 5.5 ± 5.4 years those without latex allergy. Of the 17 patients who tested positive, 11 (64.7 percent) had elevated serum IGE levels, compared with 14 with 14 of the 40 patients (35 percent) who tested negative

Safe, Latex-Free Condoms: Ending an Unpleasant Allergy Reaction?
By Anne Scheck, Medical Writer

After all, would someone who wore a latex condom suspect the bad component in the health was to blame for an itchy or painful reaction? That a person might decide against using that kind of protection in the future, he suggested. The same probably is someone who has a reaction after coming in contact with any latex product, from baby's pacifier a pair of dish gloves. But would it help to avoid all things latex "Physicians ought to thinking possibility," Dr Levy asserted. Not -So-Safe Sex Before staring his study, Dr

Levy and his colleagues surveyed a group of latex-sensitive individuals about when and how their reactions occurred. Most of the 94 men and women in the survey reaction having had an allergic reaction, including a "somatic episode" like severe breathing difficulty, immediately after using a latex condom.

In a study done in France, Dr. Levy and his colleagues found a safe alternative for those who avoid latex: "de-proteinized" condoms, which are marketed in several European countries. (The special chemical process, the protein in condoms is neutralized so that the latex derivative harmless to sensitive individuals.) These condoms did not cause a single bad reaction in men and women who previously had suffered ill effect from condom use. He added. However, several study participants did suffer the same kind of reaction they had previously experience condoms when they were exposed to other latex objects (like gloves), he observed.

It is in everything from condoms to birthday balloons-but for some people; it is a deadly allergen. Do not assume you are immune. By Susan Ferraro

It is in everything from condoms to birthday balloons - but for some people, it is a deadly allergen. Don't assume you're immune

Marion Ronee Daney

HERE'S THE RUB

New York Dailey News by Susan Ferraro

Once there was a young couple in love. One thing led to another, and "things progressed as they might when people really like each other," says Dr. Lise Borel, a health activist. Then "During intercourse, she suddenly can't breathe," continues Borel, who heard the story firsthand from the young woman. "He realized - 'Omigod, what is this? She's really in trouble!'" Gasping, the woman told her lover she might be having an allergic reaction to something at dinner. Frantic, he threw on his clothes and called 911. Paramedics took the woman to the hospital, and an alert doctor sent her to an allergen-free examining area. It was only later, after treating her, that he identified the allergen - the latex in her lover's condom

"It could have been death by condom," says Borel, who heads ELASTIC, the Education for Latex Allergy Support Team and Information Coalition. Even treating the patient was a problem - the reuse squad had latex gloves and tubing, all potential killers if you're allergic

What's a latex-allergic lover to do? You're damned if you don't use condoms- they're the foundation of safer sex, the best all-around protection against pregnancy and sexually transmitted disease.

Can Pacifiers and Diapers Trigger Allergies in Infants?
NEW YORK Rueters Health, September 30, 1999

In this case report, a 3 month-old girl developed a persistent cough, which got progressively worse in severity and became more nagging during the night, causing frequent awakenings. Since birth, she had used a rubber pacifier, especially during sleep. From her birth, she had used a rubber pacifier during the day and at night. Venuta and colleagues write, "When the rubber pacifier was replaced with a silicon one the cough disappeared," they note. She also had a history of rash on her scalp and around the diaper area. At 11 months, skin prick tests showed an allergy to natural rubber. The authors recommend that latex allergy be considered in infants with a persistent coughs who use rubber pacifiers.

Dr. Kenneth Kim said, "This is a very interesting case study," a latex expert in long Beach California. I offer this tip for parents that think their children may be allergic to latex. If your child is in a daycare center, Workers may wear latex gloves and when they change their diapers, When the workers hold up their ankles, so if it looks like your child's ankles are red, this may be a subtle sign of latex allergy,' he notes.

"As a general rule, **don't be paranoid**, but think about such subtle clues to latex allergy," he says.

Pacifiers Do Have A Positive Side
The Use Of Pacifiers and SIDS
Allergy 1999; 54:1007 Reuter Limited Copyright 1999

A Scientific study carried out by the University of Auckland, New Zealand (Mitchell)
Caused by the following

A scientific study carried out by the University of Auckland, New Zealand (Mitchell 1993 came to following Conclusion: The association between pacifier use and SIDS was investigated in 485 deaths due to SIDS in the post-neonatal age group and compared with 1800 control infants. Pacifier use in the two-week period before death was less in cases of SIDS than in the last two weeks in the control group. Use of a pacifier in the last sleep for cases of SIDS was significantly less than in the control group. It was concluded that pacifier use may protect against SIDS, but this observation needed to be repeated before pacifiers could be recommended for this purpose. However, the results of an English study, which was presented at the SIDS-Congress in Washington in June 1996, pointed in the same direction. This conformational study has just been published (Fleming 1996). It showed that the SIDS risk could be reduced by about 60% with pacifier use. Studies from Scandinavia and Chicago come to a similar conclusion, but they have yet to publish.

For more information about SIDS, please contact your local SIDS association, i.e. the American SIDS Institute (http;//www.sids.org/) or MAM Vienna.

How could a pacifier protect against SIDS?

In SIDS cases a vacuum might occur in pharynx, pulling the tongue back a blocking the airways. A pacifier may prevent the tongue sealing the airway. Pacifier use is relatively uncommon in New Zealand and if it was confirmed to have a protective effect, its promotion could reduce the number of deaths from SIDS by about 50%.

The Food Allergy & Anaphylaxis, Network Food Allergy News

How a Child Might Describe a Reaction

Children have unique ways of describing their experiences and perceptions, including allergic reactions. Time can be lost when adults do not immediately recognize that a reaction is occurring or do not understand what the children might be telling them.

These Are Examples Of What A Child Might Use To Describe A Reaction

Sometimes children, especially very young ones, will put heir hands in their mouth, or pull or scratch at their tongues, in response to a reaction. Children's voices may change (become hoarse or squeaky), and they may slur their words.

If your suspect your child is having an allergic reaction, follow your doctor's instructions.

- This food is too spicy.
- My tongue is hot (or burning).
- It feels like something is poking my tongue.
- My tongue (or mouth) itches.
- It (my tongue) feels like there is hair on it.
- My mouth feels funny.
- There's a frog is my throat.
- There's something stuck in my throat.

- My tongue feels full (or heavy).
- My lips feel tight.
- It feels like there are bugs in there (to describe itchy ears).
- It {my throat} feels thick.
- It feels like a bump is on the back of my tongue {throat}.

Allergy Hazard

Growing number of health care workers developing dangerous reaction to latex

The Patroito Ledger Tues, April 1, 1997

By Liz Kowalczyk

Doctors at South Shore Hospital in Weymouth weren't sure what was wrong when Barbara Bezanson started wheezing on the operating table. However, before long it was something serious. As soon as she arrived in the recovery room, her blood pressure plummeted. She was no longer just wheezing, but gasping for air, Bezanson, 48 of Weymouth, was going into shock. Her doctors put her on a respirator and desperately tried to figure out what was wrong. They checked for internal bleeding Negative. They searched for a drug allergy. Nothing. Then Bezanson's husband mentioned that latex gloves made her hands itch. The catheter doctors had inserted into her wound was made of the same material. She was having a severe reaction to latex. She didn't know it until the anesthesia wore off, but Benzanson had become one of the growing numbers of health care workers with serious and sometimes life-threatening allergies to latex. The natural rubber in not only found in surgical gloves, but in hundreds of household products and medical supplies. Many Massachusetts hospitals have started buying non-latex alternatives and set up "latex-free" or "latex-safe" operating rooms

Marion Ronee Daney

Is It Possible to get reactions from Tires, Asphalt, and Paving? Paving, Asphalt, Tires, and Latex Allergies: What Is The Relationship?

Latex Allergy News: Introductory Issue 1997

If you are a latex allergy victim, it is certainly possible. The Asphalt is combined with ground up tires in the paving process, which contains natural rubber. Since 1960's the recycle is in the United States, recycling tires has been used to reinforce asphalt for our roads. The components contained natural rubber, styrene-butadiene rubber (SBR), and butyl rubber. The process for paving is rubber, either in the form of ground up tires or as powdered devulcanized rubber, is added to each of the layers. Furthermore, there are no specific data concerning the exact level of natural rubber proteins in tires or rubberized asphalt. It is possible that high temperatures used in the mixing of the asphalt denature rubber proteins. Latex allergens have been found in tire dust, roadside dust and air samples from the Los Angeles areas. Tires contain natural rubber in two forms: Latex (1.4 percent proteins) and as dry sheet rubber (2.2 percent proteins).

- **Interliners** - Natural rubber is blended with butyl and SBR rubbers
- **Tire Carcass** - Natural rubber is used almost exclusively.
- **Side Walls** - Natural rubber is blended with butyl and SBR and EPDM rubbers
- **Tread cap** - Natural rubber is blended with butyl and SBR rubbers
- **Tread** - SBR is used almost exclusively

Paving with rubberized asphalt consists of the following four steps or layers

Asphalt concrete hot mixes, stress-absorbing membrane interlayer (SAMI), stress-absorbing membrane (SAM) or seal coat, and joint and crack sealers.

Therefore, Victims of latex protein hypersensitivity should avoid areas that are being paved or roofed when asphalt is being used. The airborne particles of natural latex proteins emitted in these processes are known to cause reactions in latex allergic individuals.

HOW CAN A CHILD LIFE BE DISRUPTED?

A Child's Perspective By Douglas, Pennsylvania

I am six years old and have Spina Bifida, because of that, I was told to not touch latex. It is boring to not be able to play with latex "cause lots of things are made of latex. It makes me mad that I can't chew gum especially.

When I was sick with diarrhea and had to wear diapers, I got big red marks where the elastic touched. Last fall when my dad spread sealer on our driveway, I work up sick in the night with croup. The doctor gave me a Proventil inhaler I can use now. When I get "raspy". When I get really "raspy" I have to take Albuterol syrup, it tastes yucky and it makes my hand shake. I try to be real careful and not to touch latex, but some things I don't know. I had the principal at school call the manufacturer before I would go on the new gym floor because it was spongy feeling and I was afraid. The gym teacher had to get a different ball for me. My classroom has vinyl gloves in it and I wear them when we finger paint. The teacher finds something different that the eraser dinosaurs for me to use. I do O.K. on the playground because the part that is rubber touches my hinny over clothes and not my hand

When I have birthday parties and kids give me gum, I give it to my big sister. We can't play balloon games or have them for decorations. My friends at church and kindergarten are learning about latex because of me. I remind my teacher, therapists, and sometimes my mommy to check if something is latex to keep me safe.

Marion Ronee Daney

Latex Hazards

We work with latex- But are you at Risk?

Children and Latex

In the pediatric population, as many as 250,000 children might have some degree of latex sensitivity and al least 100,000 are at serious risk when they have an operation in the presence of latex products. Children with spinal bifida are the single group with the highest incidence of latex allergy (65%).

Serious Eye injuries Associated with Water

There was a study in the May issue of Ophthalmology warns that water balloons launched by slingshots can inflict vision and life-threatening injuries. With maximum forces similar to those of rifle bullets, water balloon projectiles can perforate a cornea, rupture an eye globe, and /or fracture the bony orbit of an eye. Study author John D. Bullock, MD from Wright State University School of Medicine (Dayton, Oho) and his colleagues determined the kinetic energies of launched water balloons Maximum kinetic energies. Generated using slingshots were 176 to 245 joules in experimental studies and 141 to 232 joules in theoretical studies.

To further demonstrate the impact of these toys, researchers launched a water balloon at a stationary watermelon 20 feet away. When hit by the balloon traveling at 40 meters per second, with a kinetic energy of 240 joules, the watermelon exploded.

"These energies are comparable to or greater than kinetic energies experienced with variety of object well known to cause serious ocular injury, including some rifle bullets,"Author said. The authors also describe seventeen cases of patients with water balloon-related eye injuries. Specific eye injuries sustained by the patients ranged from traumatic cataract, retinal hemorrhages, and macular whole formation to eyelid lacerations and bony orbital wall fractures.

Authors concluded that launched water balloons represent a serious threat to vision. "It remains the responsibility of health care professionals to publicize such dangers, especially to parents who, presumable, have some influence over the purchase of such items," they said. "Indeed, the medical profession, legal profession, government, insurance industry, and general public should be aware of the enormous dangers proposed by the use of these elastic slingshots that are advertised, improperly, as "toys.""

Latex gloves hand health workers a growing worry
AMERICAN MEDICAL NEWS, Oct 13, 1997 v40 n38 pl (2)
By Margaret Veach

Seventeen years ago, Dale Long, DO, thought he was allergic to the powder inside latex surgical gloves. "Whenever anyone in the OR would put on or remove their gloves, that powder would fly, and I'd start to wheeze," he said. "I'd have to hold my breath. I got to where I could hold it for three minutes by the OR clock." Though eventually diagnosed with latex allergy, Dr Long managed to continue working for a while "by shooting up with epinephrine every 15 minutes" whenever he was at the hospital. No longer able to practice in a health care facility, he is now the medical director at a prison.

"It's the most embarrassing thing that's ever happened to me - to have to face the limitation," said Dr. Long, a general practitioner in Terre Haute, Ind. In 1988, Barbara Zucker-Pinchoff, MD, went into anaphylactic shock during the C-section delivery of her second child. She thought she was allergic to the Fentanyl used in the epidural, but an allergy to latex was diagnosed two years later. Unwilling to stop working, she hoped that taking medication and avoiding latex as much as possible would be enough to bring her allergy under control. Despite those precautions, she went into anaphylactic shock on the job six months ago and is now on total disability. Both physicians are allergic to natural rubber latex. Exactly how many of these workers are physicians are not known. Latex-sensitively, doctors have been reluctant to discuss their condition for several reasons. They are primarily afraid of losing their job, but also concerned about being stigmatized or thought of as a quitter.

In August, Dr. Zucker-Pinchoff established Physicians Against Latex Sensitization - PALS - a forum for physicians living with latex allergies as well as those concerned about stopping the increase in latex sensitization.

IN MEMORY OF:
Lt Hal Henderson (May 19, 1957 - August 29, 1997)

Education for Latex Allergy / Support Team & Information Coalition

Lieutenant Harold R. "Hal" Henderson, RN, BSN, CEN, TNCC. NC USN/RET, 40, of San Diego, California, died Friday, August 27, 1997, at the Balboa Naval Hospital. Lieutenant Henderson, who had been in ill health for some time as the result of respiratory and cardiac complications associated with latex allergy, suffered a massive heart attract. Full life support was removed at 2:15PM, Pacific Time. Hal worked tirelessly as a military liaison for ELASTIC Inc. His efforts to bring the issue of latex allergy to the attention of the Armed Services, with special attention to Navy, Veteran's Affairs and members of the California Congress; Randy "duke"Cunninham (51st District) and Bob Filner (50th District) resulted in a new awareness of the seriousness and the potential for progression of this condition. He gave support and information to military personnel who had developed allergy.

Hal' many successes will continue to receive attention; his spirit of public service is one to admired and emulated. He wanted so much to prevent others from having to go through the same needless loss of career, health and self-esteem that he did. Hal, the members of ELASTIC, trust your wish: to prevent others from suffering from latex allergy, as you have, will be granted. It is our pledge to continue your work, to continue to increase awareness, inform and educate. Perhaps your tragic and needless death will open the eyes of those who doubt, maybe this new-found awareness and a nudge from an angel or two, will allow your wish to be become reality. Lieutenant Henderson; a soldier on earth, now a soldier of God. Hal Henderson; son to Mary Ann, loving husband to Christine, devoted father to Cara Jo, Brandon Paul and Hal Jr., step-father to Nathaniel and Matthew, steadfast friend to so many, ER and ICU nurse; saving lives and safeguarding the health of countless patients, now, a guardian angel, watching from the heavens.

Hal, you are sorely missed, but your spirit and light will always be present in our

Fatal Latex Allergy
The Journal of Allergy and Clinical Immunology
March 2001, part 1 * Volume 107 * Number 3

Here we report the first case in which latex allergy had been confirmed before the fatal reaction, contact with a latex-containing agent immediately before the fatal reaction has been established, and the progression of symptoms and autopsy, findings are consistent with those of an anaphylactic death.

The deceased was a 28-year woman who had been investigated for allergy at the age of 23 years because of asthma and severe allergic reactions to nuts, with positive skin prick test responses to inhalant allergens (house dust mite, cat and dog), and nuts (strongest to Brazil nut but also to peanut, almond, and hazelnut). She was advised on proper control of the asthma and trained how to self-inject epinephrine. She was last noted to have hand eczema and skin irritation from wearing rubber gloves; a skin prick test result for latex was strongly positive. She was five detailed advice and written instructions on latex avoidance. She continued to experience significant symptoms from her asthma and other allergies and had emergency hospital treatment of an acute allergic reaction after eating. ON the day of her death, she had active eczema on her hands but had had no recent attracts of asthma. She thought not to have eaten any food to which she was allergic, and her stomach was empty at autopsy. She had hair extensions bonded with adhesive applied to a 5-cm diameter area of scalp previously affected by eczema, active the eczema had been before application of the adhesive. This adhesive was subsequently found to contain latex, to have caused reactions in latex sensitive patients, and to carry a warning that if should not but used if latex allergy was suspected. It is thought that she had never previous used this adhesive. Within 5 minutes, she reported that her scalp was itching; the woven hairs were removed, and an attempt was made to be off the adhesive. She took chlorpheniramine by mouth, but the uticaria spread and facial angioedema developed. She used her salbutamol inhaler, but her difficulty breathing rapidly became severe. She did not use the epinephrine injector that was in her handbag, immediately after her collapse, a paramedic intubated her, but attempts at resuscitation, including repeated does of epinephrine, were unsuccessful. It had been suggested that treatment with epinephrine within 30 minutes after the start of the reaction. As with other cases of fatal anaphylaxis reported recently, it is not certain that earlier treatment would have been successful. Autopsy reveled changes consistent with a severe allergic reaction, including severe periorbital and laryngeal edema with severe swelling of the lips and tongue and mucus plugging of the bronchia with mucosal edema; there was mediation emphysema. Serum from the autopsy was tested and found to have IgE antibodies to latex (8KU$_A$/L, Pharmacia Cap test) and a marginally elevated mast cell tryptase level (15*5$_1$ug/L, Pharmacia Cap test); tryptase levels may not be raised in acute allergic deaths with a major asthmatic component. The prevalence of latex allergy varies from less than 1% in the general population to as high as 12% among health care staff who routinely wear latex gloves; most of those with positive allergy test results have only mild symptoms on exposure. Anaphylactic reactions to latex affect only a small fraction of those with latex allergy, but because there is no way of accurately forecasting which of those with latex allergy may be affected, all those with histories of reactions or strongly positive allergy test responses for latex allergy must be advised about latex avoidance. This case demonstrates the dangers of less obvious sources of latex allergen and highlights the need for more effective training in the use of self-injected epinephrine. `

Laying Off Latex

The Publication of Alumni Association of New Jersey Dental School
By Sheila Smith Noonan

Dr. Ellen Patterson (92) wouldn't dream of working on patients without protective gloves, this was her nightmare. Dr. Patterson is allergic to latex. Her reaction was so severe that in April 1996 she opened a "latex-safe" practice in Fair Haven, New Jersey. It was either that, she says, or stops practicing dentistry. The first hint of this career-threatening problem surfaced when Dr. Patterson was working as a dental assistant while an undergraduate at Rutgers College. That's when she first noticed a rash on her hands "I thought nothing of it," Like everyone else, I assumed it was powder in the gloves, and tried different brands." By chance, she found that vinyl gloves weren't as irritating, but she didn't make an all -out effort to avoid latex. During dental school, a troubling problem reemerged for Dr. Patterson. She had asthma as a child, but went without an attack for many years; in fact, she ran cross-county in high school and enjoyed running. Now the asthma was back, and Dr. Patterson was using her inhaler very hour, much more frequently than the recommended one -to-four hours. She avoided latex gloves while a dental student, but in retrospect, Dr. Patterson believes the airborne latex dust from her classmates; gloves triggered the asthma. Dr. Patterson's most serious latex reaction came during her residency at Robert Wood Johnson University Hospital. As she prepared to assist oral surgeons with a procedure, she took a pair of gloves that the package label claimed was "for hands allergic to late," and gowned up. "Soon after, I didn't understand why my hands itched or why I was sneezing into my make," she says. "I went to a non-sterile are, took off the gloves and found my hands had swollen twice their size. I tried to go unnoticed, but he anesthesiologist asked what was wrong, and I told him I had latex allergies." Now, Dr. Patterson's throat was closing off, and she was going into anaphylactic shock. The anesthesiologist administered epinephrine, Benadryl, and steroids. When doctors measured her oxygen saturation level, it was worse than the original patient's by six points. By now, Dr. Patterson became an associate at one of the offices where she had been a dental assistant. Health wise, she was not doing wee. "Five minutes after I came into the offices. I would have an asthmatic reaction," she says. "I used my inhaler every hour and took antihistamines so I could work Dr. Patterson know she needed to avoid latex, but it wasn't until attending a national support group, Education for Latex Allergy Support Team and Information Coalition, or Elastic, that she realized how others' use of the product affected her through the airborne particles. Therefore, she asked her employer to adapt their office to be as latex-safe as possible. He both a filtration unit, which helped somewhat, and partly converted to non-latex gloves, but sometimes-latex gloves were used, and Dr. Patterson's problems continued after not working on Friday, she came into the office Saturday and used the computer. "I must have brushed my hair from my eyes, because within minutes both of my eyes were completely swelled shut." I gave my self of epinephrine, but appointments still were canceled, "recalls Dr. Patterson. With latex, there's a phenomenon known as touch transfer, where the dust settles everywhere. The other dentist must have been wearing latex gloves; she believes, took them off and then used the computer inadvertently contaminating it. Dr. Patterson says she "had a lot of soul searching to do." In late 1995 she left the practice and and decide whether to quit dentistry, start a new practice, or purchase an existing one. She chose the latter, and because the previous dentist used latex, had the office thoroughly cleaned before opening her doors in April 1996. Dr. Patterson describes her office as latex safe instead of latex free because she says it's impossible to claim the entire product is eliminated. There is latex tubing in some of the office's larger equipment and the diaphragm under her computer keyboard is made of natural rubber latex. Still, she uses place syringes and purchases local anesthetic in individual glass ampules. Her gloves are either nitrile, which she prefers and uses most often, or vinyl. Nitrile offers better puncture-resistance than latex and is not worn down by glutaraldehyde, she says. Many studies have faulted vinyl for it's tearing, but Dr. Patterson says its use, for her, is procedure-dependent. "When I wear vinyl gloves for 10 to 20 minutes. I feel I'm afforded the protection I'm looking for," she says. As for tactile sensitivity, Dr. Patterson says nitrile and vinyl perform as well for her as latex. About 10 percent of Dr. Patterson's patients are allergic to latex. Many, have with delayed dental care because of their allergies or asked dentists not to wear latex gloves and been refused. Latex-safe dental offices are so difficult to find, one patient comes from Boston. "Unfortunately, I don't think many dentists understand the airborne component of latex allergies," says Dr. Patterson. "Their resistance to latex-safe offices isn't from lack of compassion. They just don't grasp the full effects of latex allergies. However, I'm hopeful dentistry will come through on this important matter. Dentist are traditionally prevention oriented, and this is a very prevention-oriented issue." Dr. Patterson's heath has improved since she opened her latex-safe office, although she still has avoided latex product in all aspects of her life. Balloons are taboo ('I see balloons as some people view guns-extremely dangerous'), and she phones restaurants ahead to find out whether food preparation workers use latex gloves. Professionally, Dr. Patterson is coming into her own. There were many times, she admits, when she felt like walking away from dentistry. But when she treats patients with latex allergies, it' as though she has answered a calling. "I know how lucky I am to be healthy and practicing dentistry," she says. "After I treat someone with this allergy, I know it' what I need to do.

Local Woman Lives In Fear
The Newport Daily News Friday, April 9, 1999
By Terrence Synnott, Daily News Staff

Vallarie E. Mayville of Middletown has a potentially fatal allergy to latex. Because of that, she wants the town to eliminate latex balloon and gloves from the school, or she will educate her children at home. In addition, it's unclear when, and if, they will return. Until her demands are met. For the past month, Mayville, who has a potentially fatal allergy to latex, but been pushing for a school-wide ban on latex balloons. When has called the superintendent. She has called School Committee. She has had her control send a letter to school officials attesting of the surety of her condition. She has had no luck. Mayville said her children's exposure to latex at school puts her life at risk. Allergic reactions to latex range from hives to asthma to anaphylactic shock and possibly death. A former dental assistant, Mayville believes repeated exposure to the substance caused the allergy. Inhaling trace amounts of latex - which can be carried home on the children's clothes - can trigger allergic reactions, she said. When a reaction is coming on, Mayville first gets a metallic taste in her mouth. Her eyes water. Her voice cracks because of swelling in her throat. She gets hives and begins to sweat. "And there's a sense of doom like I'm dying," Mayville said. The news of her condition hit her hard. "My allergist (Dr. Anthony R. Ricci) was looking at my charts and he said, "Well, you better quit your job. You had better change your major Mayville said. "I thought my life was over or at least the life I had known to that point." The family is constantly looking out of products containing latex. Her husband, Bob, a Portsmouth EMT, must shower at the Portsmouth fire station before returning home. Her children call home from school if they encountered latex products and tell their mother to have a change of clothes ready for them. When they arrive home, they immediately strip down to their underwear and head for the shower, someone starts a load off laundry. Mayville's fear of latex also keeps her from leaving the house. Her husband does most of the grocery shopping and he takes the children doctor appointments and on most other trips. Mayville fights back tears as she talks about the change and impact they have had on her family. "You go from bring a really active, outgoing, fun person to being a shadow of who you once were," she said. She described the months following her diagnosis as a difficult time, one mainly spent in bed crying. In recent months, Mayville said, she has started to take more control of her life. She spends May hours each day on her computer, reading about latex allergy and communicating with others who have the condition. Mayville feels a sense of empowerment she originally lost when she lost and when she was forced to quit he According to statistics from the U.S. Department of Health and Human Services, reports about of the general population and prevalence of latex allergy vary greatly About 1 percent to 6 percent about 8 percent to 12 percent of regularly exposed health care worker have some type of sensitivity to latex.

Iowa

Pat: ELASTIC
Education for Latex Allergy/ Support Team & Information Coalition
This is a letter appeared in the March 1996 issue of Latex Allergy News.

Debi - I know that you receive so many letters full of anger and despair. I wanted to write a really upbeat, cheery letter, but like so many before me, there is a downside before the uphill struggle. My name is Pat Lawson; I live in Council Bluff, Iowa. I was a Certified Surgical Technician from 1975, I have a latex allergy. I quit my job (reluctantly) in Janua4ry 1993 due to numerous unexplained illnesses and absenteeism. I was viewed by co=workers as lazy, stressed out or a hypochondriac. I was told in 1992 that I had occupational asthma, but never once did the words "latex" escape my allergist's lip. It wasn't until a friend attending a workshop and I saw Carol Brown (ELASTIC Nebraska) that I had any idea of what I was experiencing. Even after the diagnosis was made, I was in denial. I kept up the pretense that one day I would return to the OR. In September of 1995, my allergist looked me in the eye and said "NEVER AGAIN "! The pain, the rage, the frustration. Like an alcoholic, I needed to hit rock bottom before I could start the healing cycle, and boy, did I ever plunge to the bottom. Do not worry about me. I climbed out of the emotional low with vengeance. Rejection does strange thing to our minds, and it made me mad as hell! I'm mad that I have this allergy, I'm mad I allowed people to humiliate me, and I'm mad I allowed people to humiliate me, and I'm mad I can not continued in the job I loved and spent and spent to many years doing well. What has because of ignorance? I am so frustrated! The lack of education caused me to loose my career and life style, and now I am fighting back! I gave my first in-service yesterday, and I have one or two more scheduled, I am a woman with a mission. Education! I have already spoken to Lise Borel and watch out Iowa, here I come!!! I want to thank you and everyone involved in Latex Allergy education. You gave me the courage to stand up and fight for myself. By having one friend hearing an in-service, you and Carol saved my life. I can never repay you, but I will do all I can to try to save one more person from having to experience what I have been through I know this is long; I apologize, but it sis so nice to be able to vent and to say "God! I am glad I am alive", Thank you.

Hospital Are Saying No To Latex Balloons
Latex Balloons Banned From Hospital
Focus on the Law, June 1999 Volume 21, #5

No Latex Balloons, Please! That is the new sign being posted through out hospitals in the United States and Canada. The hospitals are adopting a "no latex balloons' policy in an effort to reduce their patients" and staff members' exposure to latex. Keeping latex balloons off the pediatric floors at hospital is becoming a major priority. People who had had spinal or bladder problems as children and used catheters, or people who have had multiple surgeries, may be greater risk.

Hospital Changes Policy to Address Latex Allergies
Breaking News
American City Business Journals Inc. February 4, 2000

Niagara Falls Memorial Medical Center is now prohibiting the use of latex balloons at the center to ensure the safety of patients, visitors and staff who may be allergic to latex. The amount of latex exposure needed to produce symptoms is unknown, but the symptoms can begin within minutes or take hours after exposure.

Hospitals Striving To Be Latex-Free
*Balloons And Glover Are Among Products That Might Cause Allergic Reactions
The Morning Call November 16, 1999 By Diane Marczely Cimpel

The fistful of colorful balloons you thought would cheer up a sick friend or relative in the hospital? Latex can make people allergic to it sick. Because of that, some hospital won't even let balloons made with the rubber in the front door. That is new policy at St. Luke's Quakertown Hospital in Allentown and at Easton Hospital. Latex can spark a variety of reactions in those who are allergic, from a mild rash where the latex touches the skin to airway constriction, which can hamper breathing according to Ellen Reker, Vice President of patient services at St. Luk's Quakertown. "That's relatively uncommon but because of the nature and severity of the reaction, it's incumbent upon us to limit the possibility of that happening," Reker said. In the past week, St. Luke's Quakertown instituted the latex balloon ban. Signs will go up alerting visitors and florists are being notified.

Latex balloons. . Leave'em at home please!
The Finley Hospital March 2000

There are a growing number of people who are sensitive and /or allergic to the latex contained in items such as balloons. In addition, it is not a laughing matter. Therefore, latex balloons are no longer permitted as patient gifts at The Finley Hospital. The ban is not meant to discourage well 'wishers. Latex balloons are dangerous because they contain large amounts of the allergen protein as well as powder, which absorb latex proteins. When a balloon is inflated, deflated popped, or handled, the powder is free to contaminate the air. If a latex-allergic individual inhales the powder, respiratory distress and /or anaphylactic shock can occur.

If you would like to bring balloon to a patient, Mylar or foil balloon are safe choices.

Clinton Hospital Bans Latex Balloons
QUAD-CITY TIMES-December 8, 1999 Bt Ross Bielama

They have two choices: leave the balloons with a volunteer greeter or take them back to their car. The hospital has instituted an outright ban on latex balloons to protect patient, employees and staff room potential health problems caused by allergies to latex. "We haven't done this because we want to be mean," said Gina Schwartz, employee health coordinator at Mercy. "We're doing this for safety." A volunteer who says greets unsuspecting visitors who want to cheer up a patient with a balloon bouquet: "I'm sorry. We cannot allow the balloon to go up to a patient's room. The hospital gift shop also has stopped selling latex balloons, but does offer Mylar balloon, which do not cause allergy problems, Schwartz said. "We sent letter to all the vendors—flower shops, grocery stores—that we were doing this," she said. The rubber leaches into the cornstarch, and then is spread into the air and on doorknobs and other surfaces. The hospital's Latex Committee previously prompted the hospital to switch to non-powdered latex gloves, which eliminates the airborne particles. Now, the committee agreed that latex balloons should go, too.

Latex gloves, balloons and other products typically have a light dusting of cornstarch – the whit powder you find on hands and lips when blowing up many balloons – to prevent the rubber from sticking together, Schwartz said. The rubber leaches into the cornstarch – a swelling of the airways that can lead to be fatal.

Anaphylaxis Reports

Departments of Anesthesiology, Surgery, Division of Pediatric Surgery and Nursing
University of Virginia Health Sciences Center

Anaphylaxis under general anesthesia is rare, estimated to occur in 1: 10,000 -1: 25.000 anesthetic and it is most commonly associated with the administration of antibiotic (1). Introperative anaphylaxis to latex product has also been described (2,3)). Patients with frequent exposure to latex product are considered at high risk. "High - risk patients" include children requiring frequent urogentiaital instrumentation, e.g. children with myelodysplastic syndromes, spinal bifida or meiogomeelocele (3,4). We describe a child with an intraoperative anaphylactic reaction to latex that presented as a sudden loss of end -tidal carbon dioxide on the capnograph. This case differs from most cases described in the literature in this child had no previous history of latex allergy, did not fall in the high - risk group of latex sensitive patients and had multiple exposures to latex in the preoperative period without obvious adverse effects.

Case Report

A six-year-old boy with a history of Hirshcsprung's disease was scheduled for exploratory laparotomy for a small bowel obstruction. He had undergone three previous bowel resections without anesthetic problems during his first year of life. Postoperative sepsis and a prolonged stay in the pediatric intensive care unit complicated the second operation. He was taking Ritalin for attention deficit disorder and had no other medical problems or known allergies.

An intravenous catheter was placed and the patient had been rehydrated with normal saline solution prior to his arrival to the operating suite. Midazolam, 2mg was administered IV in the holding area. An ECG, pulse oximeter and blood pressure cuff were applied in the operating room. His initial heart rate (HR) was 140bpm; blood pressure (BP) was 110/70 mmHg and oxygen saturation (02 sat) was 100%, General anesthesia was induced with the intravenous administration of sodium thiopental (125mg) and 20mg of rocuronium was administered IV to facilitate endotracheal intubations with an uncuffed 5 mm endotracheal tube (ETT). The breath sounds were clear to auscultation and an air leak around the ETT was present at 18 cm water pressure. Capnography confirmed endotracheal intubations and the initial end tidal pCO_2 (Et pCO_2) was 45 mmHg. Immediately after intubations, vital signs were as follows: BP 114/68 mmHg and the O2 Sat 100%. Fentanyl, 20 mcg was administered IV and general anesthesia was maintained with 1 - 1.2% isoflurane, 50% air and 50% oxygen.

Ten minutes after induction and five minutes after incision, during dissection of bowel adhesions, the Et pCO_2 abruptly decreased to 0. Breath sounds were absent. Direct laryngoscopy confirmed endotracheal placement of the ETT. Manual ventilation proved unsuccessful in generating breath sound or and Et pCO2 on the capnograph. The O2 Sat at this point was 100%, BP 118 / 64 mmHg, HR 123. The patient was reintubated with 5.5 mm cuffed ETT in the hope that effective ventilation would be achievable with higher airway pressures. However, reintubation did not improve ventilation in spite of higher airway pressures, and it was suspected that severe bronchospam was responsible for the sudden absence of Et pCO2. At this point aerosolized albuterol was administered via the ETT. BP, HR and O2 Sat weren't changed appreciably from previous values. Repeated administration of aerosolized albuterol and the administration of glycopyrrolate, 0.4mg IV, did not improve ventilation (5). Subsequently the O2 Sat decreased to 65%, the patient became hypotensive (40mmHg systolic) and bradycardia developed (HR 58). Epinephrine was administered in repeated doses (100 mcg IV total dose) and BP was restored. Approximately 30 seconds after the administration of the last dose of epinephrine, ventilation and oxygenation improved. The O2 Sat returned to 100%, and the patient was manually ventilated until at Et pCO2 of 35 mmHg was achieved. At this point flushing of the patients face, trunk and upper was noted, and 4 mg dexamethasone as well as 20 mg diphenhydramine was administered IV. A second reaction occurred when the surgeons remedy the operation, requiring further resuscitation with epinephrine. Since bother episodes occurred during extensive bowel manipulation, we considered the administered, as described previously by Latson et al (6). Simultaneously one of the operating room nurses suggested the child may have a latex allergy, and the surgeons changed to latex - free gloves minimal wheezing was audible, and the O2 Sat immediately after extubation was 97% on 4 L oxygen delivered by face tent.

When questioned postoperatively, the patient's mother related a history of face and arm flushing over the previous year whenever blowing up balloons or when being examined in the physician's office with gloves. However, he had never developed cardio respiratory difficulties.

A Radioallergosorbent (RAST) assay was performed and was strongly positive for latex antibodies, which confirmed the suspicion of a latex allergy. The child was given a medical alert bracelet prior to leaving the hospital.

In this case the preoperative interview and examination did I not suggest that the child had a latex sensitivity? Additionally, the child did not fall into the high-risk group of patients described above; both factors contributed to delayed diagnosis of latex allergy. Upon loss of the ET pCO2, correct ETT placement was confirmed and the patient was re - incubated with a cuffed

ETT Abdominal retractors placed by the surgeon were initially thought to have decreased the patient's pulmonary compliance, and we thought that delivering larger airway pressures through a cuffed ETT However, his intervention proved to unsuccessful and bronchospasm as the cause for the poor ventilatory status was considered to be the causative factor. Anaphylaxis as the mediator was not immediately deliberated because no drugs were administered within least five minutes prior to the events. Since both episodes coincided with surgical manipulations of the mesentery, release of intestinal mediators precipitating the Mesenteric Traction Syndrome as describe during abdominal aortic aneurysm surgery was suspected (7). Anaphylaxis to latex was only considered after the second, - Fatal episode. We speculate that the prolonged intensive care unit stay after one of these previous operations may have sensitized the child to latex.

Prior to the cardiovascular collapse, our patient had multiple - exposures to latex during this hospitalizations. Immediately prior to his arrival in the operating room, our patient was handled with - continuing examination gloves. Anesthetic drug were administered through latex - containing injections ports in the IV tubing and a latex- containing rubber mask was applied to the child's face anesthetic induction. A time span of at least 15 minutes passed after induction and intubation, last through skin incision and it was not until surgical manipulation of the intestine that ventilatory insufficiency followed by cardiorespiratory collapse developed. Although the child was exposed to latex- containing products through out, massive antigen exposure from the surgical gloves delivered via the highly vascular serosal surfaces of the bowel was required to trigger the events. Once this agent load was removed and latex - free the surgeons, the patient experience n further problems, used gloves. This was in spite of the fact that latex - continuing rubber stopcocks in the IV bag and a latex - continuing breathing bag in the circle breathing system were continued to be used throughout the remainder of the case. Just like prior uneventful exposure, concurrent exposure late via a less invasive route will not guarantee the safe use of latex. The fact that latex anaphylaxis occurred only with bowel manipulation was undoubtedly important in the delayed diagnosis and delayed to proper treatment in this case.

In summary, this case illustrates a dramatic anaphylactic reaction to latex in a child without history latex allergies who does not fall in the classic "high - risk" group of children. We feel that all children with a history of multiple hospital admissions, especially if associated with prolonged intensive care, should be included in the group of potentially latex - sensitive patients.

In retrospect, history and more detailed questioning regarding reactions of the child toward exposure to latex have prevented the intraoperative events. The experience with this case led our hospital to mod operative screening to routinely include specific questions regarding a possibility of latex allergic all pediatric patients.

Natural Rubber Latex Allergy: A Potentially Disabling Epidemic
By Rochelle D. Spiker, MSW, LCSW-C
Executive Director of the Potomac Latex Allergy Association

I have a severe allergy to commonplace substance, rubber. Enough exposure to rubber could result in my going into shock or even dying if not promptly treated. When I interview for a new job I now tell my prospective employer this -in the presence of powdered latex gloves, I am 100% disabled. In the absence of powdered latex gloves, I am 0% disabled. They quickly see the value in accommodating to my disability if I am to become their employee. Unfortunately for many healthcare workers, often employers to keep the powdered latex gloves and dismiss their latex allergic employees. Natural rubber latex allergy is potentially disabling, it is also a danger to those already disabled from other sources.

I am the Executive Director of a locally based support group known as the Potomac Latex Allergy Association, here in Washington, D.C. When I talk to people about being severely allergic to rubber many roll their eyes at me as if I am insane, or laugh aloud. This allergy is no laughing matter, however. The first indication that I was latex allergic was in 1984, went to a number of physicians complaining about my symptoms, none of them properly diagnosed me as being latex allergic, and my sensitization continued. At this point in my life, I can never wear latex gloves or have any form of rubber used inside of me again. Luckily, for me there are viable alternatives. Gloves made out of nitrile afford as good a barrier protection as latex, but lack some of the durability. Polyurethane condoms do exist, bulk are less durable than latex. My place of employment has accommodated to my disability by going powder-free, so I am able to continue to work full time as a social worker. Other people with latex allergy are not as fortunate. Their employers deny that the gloves they have worn on the job have caused or contributed to their allergy. They are told they are hysterical or psychosomatic. They are forced to visit worker's compensation doctors who know little or nothing about latex allergy for a diagnosis. They are forced to take tests for the illness that have a high rate of false negatives. If they are given an incorrect diagnosis solely based on a false negative test result, they are told to return to the same environment that is making them sick, or quit. Exposed to too much aerosolize glove powder in their professions, many are suffering from occupational asthma and cardiomyopthy. Two nurses in Oregon and one in California recently died as a direct result of complications from their latex allergy. The deaths in Oregon spurred on introduction of an anti-glove powder bill in 1997, due to the influence of the Rubber Industry, that bill has been tabled. Other similar bill have been introduced in other states, all have been styled by the Rubber Industry. Despite my experience with rubber, I do not advocate that it be banned. I do advocate the banning of powdered latex gloves. Powder-free latex gloves are available on the market. I also advocate for the extensive education of all groups that are being especially marketed to by the rubber industry. Natural rubber latex products can be made safer, less allergenic and should be. It is only when the consumers unite and begin to demand just that that the current conditions will change.

Attention: Health, Industrial and forward planning editors
100,000 NHS staff allergic to gloves designed to protect
July 30, 2001

At least 100,000 NHS staff at risk from a potentially life-threatening allergy to latex could be protected if hospital and ambulances provided an alternative to the potentially deadly rubber, the TUC says in a report today (Wednesday). Providing an alternative to latex in the health service would prevent these NHS works from developing the allergy in the first place, and protect the estimated half a million people already allergic to latex. There is no way to predict how severe the reaction will be when a latex allergy sufferer comes into contact with the rubber, but people have died as a result. TUC Senior Heath and Safety Policy Officer, Owen Tudor, said: 'Latex gloves were once seen as part of the solution to occupational diseases, but now they're part of the problem. For the sake of a few pence for a pack of gloves, workers' health is being put at risk, and patient health is compromised.

Case#3

Judith Barnes worked as a State Registered Chiropodist in Lancashire. She developed Type 1 latex allergy through wearing powdered latex gloves at work in the NHS. Despite switching in wearing vinyl gloves, everyone else continued to use latex gloves, which led to more allergic reactions. I was forced to take ill-health retirement – even though I was only 34. Judith decided to sue her employer and after a long battle, lasting over three years she finally won. Her Health Trust admitted liability for causing latex allergy and made the medical environment safer. Judith feels that her life now is totally changed and now she cannot go swimming or to gym anymore. When shopping, Judith has to make it short and certain shops she has to avoid altogether. "This is not hypochondria," Judith says; 'I know how ill you feel with latex-allergy, and no matter what any doctor says, it is potentially life-threatening.'

Judith adds: 'On a hospital visit to dermatologist who was using powdered latex glove. I ended up in casualty surrounded by doctors, given oxygen, steroids and antihistamines. I have also had problems at the dentist and had to have a minor operation cancelled due to the risk of allergy in theatre.'

Case #4

Fiona McKie-Bell worked at Newcastle's Royal Victoria Infirmary where she wore latex gloves. She started to experience anaphylactic reactions to latex, which included swelling up of the face, lips and airways whist working and was eventually force into medical retirement at the age of 25. However, the pain and suffering did not stop for Fiona after retiring. She was due to have a wisdom tooth removed under local anesthetic at a large teaching hospital. Although the dentist knew she was allergic to natural rubber latex (NRL), a syringe with an NRL bung was inadvertently used, and Fiona suffered an anaphylactic reaction. She spent the next few days in the intensive treatment unit, where she had several more anaphylactic reactions. Since then she has been hospitalized 50 times in only eight months. She uses nebulised adrenaline to help her breathing and is virtually housebound.

'All this is due to ignorance, but I and many others are left with a life long allergy which money alone cannot compensate.'

Greendale Firefighter claims Disability, blaming Latex
Milwaukee-Journal Sentinel Staff
By Kenneth R. Lamke`
December 16, 1997

A Fire Department lieutenant is seeking a duty disability pension because of her sensitivity to latex, In Greendale. The Fire Chief James Strange said that presumably from the gloves she wears on the job. Strange also said that the city will not contest the case. Kowalski has been off duty since March, when she suffered what appeared to be a latex-related reaction after responding to a call said Chief James Strange.

Kowalski when to three doctors and they have found that she could no longer perform her duties

Because on her job she is, require to wear the latex gloves, Strange said. An Attorney representing Wausau Insurance Co. Joseph G. Gibart. Which covers Greendale employees, said the firm is not contesting the doctor's findings. 'According to Howard Myers, Kowalski's those findings must be confirmed by the stat Department of Employee Trust Funds. The Insurance Company Attorney, Gilbert said that while it was unusual for a case of debilitating latex sensitivity to emerge form a Fire Department. Kowalski's medical role put her in the line of work in which such allergies are most often seen Strange said that the Fire Department had already ordered non-latex gloves for its employees but added that it would be hard to accommodate Kowalski by banning all latex products, because the material is found in so much equipment.

In 1995, Kowalski, then a firefighter, filed a sex discrimination complaint against the department, saying she had been unfairly passed over for promotion in favor of less qualified males. Strange said that Kowalski was promoted to lieutenant in settlement of the complaint.

R | D Group study on 27 cases with latex allergy

Ritsuko Hayakawa*,
Research Group for New Material of Rubber Products
*Department of Environmental Dermatology, Nagoya University School of Medicine,

| @Abstract

| @ | @ To investigate the actual conditions of latex allergy in Japan and prevent recurrence and new development of latex allergy, we organized the Research Group for New Material of Rubber Products. We carried out the group study on patients with latex allergy.

The cases studied composed of 19-contact urticaria, 4-contact urticaria accompanied by contact dermatitis, 2 contact dermatitis and 2 anaphylaxis.

Nineteen subjects (90.5%) out of 21 tested showed positive results to latex specific IgE. Eight out of 21 (38.1%) had positive results to banana, 9 (42.9%) to avocado and 7 (33.3%) to kiwi specific IgE.

Eight (44.4%) of 18 also had positive result to potato and 9 (50.0%) to tomato specific IgE. As to the results of scratch testing, 17 cases out of 24 tested (70.8%) reacted positively to the extract solution of natural rubber gloves (NRG), 18 cases (75.0%) reacted positively to the extract solution of the patient's rubber gloves (LPG) and only 2 cases (8.0%) to the extract solution of low latex protein contained rubber gloves (LPG). We concluded that latex allergy is an important problem to be solved.

| @ | Key words: latex allergy, group study, natural rubber gloves, and low latex protein rubber gloves

| @ | @ Latex allergy is an important problem in medical and dental field (1-3), In the case of anaphylaxis (4), it is life threatening, In recent years, latex allergy has become a problem also in daily life

To investigate the actual conditions of latex allergy in Japan and prevent recurrence and new development of latex allergy, we organized the Research Group of New Material of Rubber Products. We carried out the group study on patients with latex allergy. Institutes participated in this study were nine University Hospitals, four General Hospitals and National Institute for Hygiene participate in this study (Table 1)

Table 1 Institutes participated

Department of Environmental Dermatology, Nagoya University School of Medicine (Nagoya University Daiko Medical Center)

Department of Dermatology, Yokohama City University Urafune Hospital
Department of Dermatology, Kansai Medical University Hospital
Department of Dermatology, Gunnma University Hospital
Department of Dermatology, Hyougo Medical College Hospital
Department of Dermatology, Aich Medical University Hospital
Department of Dermatology, Koube University Hospital
Department of Dermatology, Yamanashi Medical University Hospital

Department of Dermatology, Toho Medical University Hospital
Department of Dermatology, Koube Rousai Hospital
Department of Dermatology, Yamaguchi Red Cross Hospital
Department of Dermatology, Sakai Municipal Hospital
Department of Dermatology, Nissan Kouseikai Tamgwa Hospital
National Institute for Hygiene

@ **Subjects and Materials**

| @ | @ Twenty-seven patients with latex allergy who visited the above hospitals in 1997 were studied. The subjects were composed of 13 medical workers, 2 dental worker, 4 other workers using rubber gloves, 5 housewives and 3 others (Table **2**)

Table 2 Background of the subjects

Sex: 4 males and 21 females

Age: 22 - 46 year - old (mean age 31.3 years old)

Occupation: 14 medical workers, a dental worker, 3 other workers using rubber gloves, 5 housewives and 2 others.

A topic predisposition: positive 19 (76%), negative 6 (24)

Materials: Scratch/prick test: The extract solution of a brand of latex gloves on the market, an experimental low latex protein contained latex gloves, an ammoniated latex sheet, rubber gloves used by patients were prepared. The test solutions of banana, avocado, and kiwi were also prepared.

| @ | @ Patch testing: Thiuram mix, PPD black rubber mix, Mercapto mix, Mercapto mix, Dithiocarbamate mix an extract solution is an ammoniated latex sheet were prepared (Table 3).

Table 3 Materials of skin testing

Scratch/prick test
The extract solution of a brand of latex gloves on the market
An experimental low latex protein contained rubber gloves
An ammoniated latex sheet

Rubber gloves used by the patients
The test solutions ofbanana
Avocado
Kiwi
Patch testing
Thiuram mix, PPD black rubber mix, Mercapto mix
Dithiocarbamate mix 28 other relevant allergens
Extract solution of an ammoniated latex sheet

IgE RAST: Latex, banana, avocado, kiwi, potato and tomato were examined

| @ | @Scratch/prink test: Using PRICK-LANCETTER (1 mm spiss) with shoulders to prevent deeper penetration, we carried out the scratch or the prick test with the test materials. Readings were made after 20 and 60 minutes comparing the reaction of 1% histamine.

| @ | @patch testing: Using Finn Chamber and Scanpor tape, we performed 48-closed patch testing with test materials on the upper back of the patients.

| @ | @Readings were made at 1 and 24 hours after removals according to ICDRG recommendations.

| @ | @Usage test: If needed, after confirming no symptoms on the patient's finger, usage test with rubber gloves one finger was carried out. When the patient claimed itching, the test material was removed. Erythema and /or wheal were read as positive signs

| @ | @IgE RAST: We utilized Pharmacia CAP-RAST.

| @**Results**

| @ @Type of allergy: 19 contact urticaria, 4 contact urticaria accompanied by contact dermatitis and 2 anaphylaxis. Nineteen subjects (90.5%) out of 21 tested showed positive results to latex specific IgE. Eight out of 21 (38.1%) had positive results to banana, 9 (42.9%) to avocado and 7 (33.3%) to kiwi specific IgE.

| @ | @Eight (44.4%) of 18 also had positive results to potato and 9 (50.0%) to tomato specific IgE.

| @ | @As to the results of scratch testing, 17 cases out of 24 tested (70.8%) reacted positively to the extract solution of natural rubber gloves (NRG), 18 cases of (75.0%) reacted positively to the extract solution of the patient's rubber gloves (LRG) and only 2 cases (8.0%) to the extract solution of low latex protein contained rubber gloves (LPG). Four cases showed positive reactions by patch testing. They reacted to thiuram mix, extract solution of ammoninated latex sheet and N-Isopropyl-N'-phenyl IPPD (Table 4).

TABLE 4RESULTS OF SKIN TESTINGS

Scratch testingPositive/Tested (%)
Extract solution of natural rubber gloves (NRG):17/24 (70.8%)
Extract solution of patient's gloves (PG):18/24 (75.2%)
Extract solution of low latex protein contained : 2/25 (8.0%)
Rubber gloves (LPG)

Patch testing
Thiuram mix: 2/26 (7.7%)
N-Isopropyl-N'-phenyln IPPD: 1/26 (3.8%)
Extract solution of ammoniated latex sheet: 1/26 (3.8%)

| @ | @Twenty-seven patients with latex allergy were examined. Twenty-three patients (85.2%) were contact urticaria, and 4 of them also suffered from contact dermatitis due to latex. Seventeen cases out of 24 tested (70.8%) reacted positively to the extract solution of natural rubber gloves (NRG), 18 cases (75.0%) reacted positively to the extract solution of the patient's rubber gloves (LPG) and only 2 cases (8.0%) to the extract solution of low latex protein contained rubber gloves (LPG). We concluded that LPG is safe and useful products. Four cases showed patch test positive reactions.

| @ | @They reacted to thiuram mix, extract solution of ammoniated latex sheet and N-Isopropyl-N'-phenyl IPPD. Although not frequent type IV allergy due to latex was seen. Two cases were anaphylaxis; both experienced dyspnea, drop of blood pressure and lost of consciousness. We conclude that latex allergy is an important problem to be solved.

Marion Ronee Daney

| @References

Hayakawa R: latex contact Allergy, Evniron Dermato; 3:60-63. 1996

Sugiura M, Hayakawa R, Kato Y: A case of latex contact allergy, Environ Dermatol 3:165-169,1996

Tanaka

S, Hayakawa R. Sugiura M: A case of contact urticaria due to latex, Environ Dermato

4:225-230. 1997

Sugiura M. Hayakawa R: a Case of anaphylaxis due to latex, Environ Dermatol 4: 142-145. 1997

Update on the Law...
Latex Allergy Litigation

United States Workers' Compensation Programs are Becoming Sensitized to Latex
By Jon. L. Gelman {1}

Throughout United States, there has been a phenomenon in Workers' compensations for cases involving Latex allergy sensitivity claims. During the years between 1988 and 1995 there have been led to the reporting of 23 deaths to the Federal Drug Administration. The casual relationship between latex exposure and allergic reaction can cause anaphylactic shock. The natural latex rubber is used for so many things. Latex gloves help protect against diseases is one of the products made, which also there are over 40,000 medical, surgical and household products. There has been estimated that over 950,000 healthcare workers may become sensitized to latex protein during their careers.

There are three types of disease were considered in locating reported workers' compensation decision. 1) First type-irritant contact dermatitis involving non-allergic reactions, 80% of disease base. Between 25% and 40% of glove wearers, develop a mild irritant reaction. 2) Second type was Type IV hypersensitivity-delayed reaction, occurring several hours and possibly up to four days after re-exposure to the substance initially. 3) Third type-Type 1 hypersensitivity-is very serious, it occurs when an antigen interacts with an antibody, immediate response by the immune system that can occur within minutes or one to two hours after exposure. In addition, it can have

104

reactions: localized hives, generalized hives with facial and throat swelling, hives, swelling, hives with asthma involvement of the nose, throat, ears, and digestive tract, or a life-threatening systemic reaction, anaphylaxis.

The case law disclosure that 13 states had reported cases: Illinois, Mississippi, Minnesota, Montana, New York, Oregon, Pennsylvania, South Dakota, Texas, Vermont, Virginia, Washington, and Wisconsin. Of the 30 reported cases nationally, 21 were deemed compassable under the Workers' Compensation Acts of the various jurisdictions. The claims from the period of 1987 through 19999 demonstrate that there has been significant increase in those seeking benefits because of latex sensitivity. Since the last reported case an available for consideration was decided on June 30, 1999, estimated projections for the third and fourth quarters of 1999 were utilized. The claims seem to be clustered in various jurisdictions including Wisconsin, New York, Texas, Virginia and South Dakota. The states Wisconsin and New York demonstrated that a claim for latex sensitivity is extremely serious in nature and is indeed compassable. This significantly percentages of the claims were awarded of total and permanent disability benefits to the claimant.

A Nurse Aide was awarded total disability benefits in the state Montana by the court. She worked for the Kalispell Regional Hospital and was required to use latex gloves while working with a patient who was in isolation. When the procedure progressed, her hands swelled up and developed abdominal pain, nausea and vomiting. She was hospitalized and her physicians conducted an examination for rectal and pelvic with latex gloves, her reactions became worse. The Nurse Aide had a barium enema utilizing latex equipment for purpose of diagnosing her unexplained abdominal pain, her blood pressure began to fall and she went into anaphylactic shock. The case was very unique to the workers' compensation hearing official, her disability was so severe because of its life-threatening potential that the official stated, and "there may well be no equitable solution." She was awarded totally and permanently disabled, the court awarded a suitable housing should be located and threat a price should be reached which would allow a lump sum of advance of benefits.

In the conclusion, since the workers' compensation remedies may in fact be inadequate to monetarily compensation the petitioners, the victims of latex allergies are also filing product liability claims against the suppliers' manufacturers and distributors of latex products.

LATEX ALLERGY NEWS
Volume VI issue 5
June1999
ISSN (SSN#1084-1121)

TABLE 1
GENERAL SYMPTOMS
Type 1 (*IgE mediated*)

Runny nose	sinusitis	rash**
Shortness of breathe	asthma	purities
Sneezing	skin reactions	rhino conjunctivitis
Coughing	dyspnea	ocular itching and/or
Nasal itching	urticaria (hives)	swelling
Chest tightness	headache	angioedema
Nasal congestion	dermatitis**	
Wheezing	itching	

**Most common latex allergy symptoms

TABLE 11. SYSTEMATIC ALLERGY SYMPTOMS

Urticarcia/hives	stridor
rhino conjunctivis	laryngeal edema
Rhino rhea/clear discharge	
Angioedema (swelling)	*Cardiovacular*
Ocular	tachycardia
Edema (organ specific)	hypotension
Flushing/facial redness	arrhythmia
Shortness of breath	
Facial swelling	*Gastrointestinal*
Coughing	nausea
Fainting	vomiting
Asthma	diarrhea
Shock	abdominal cramping/pain
Wheezing	

TABLE 111. SKIN REACTIONS TO LATEX

Reaction	Response
Irritation Contact Dermatitis	red, chapped hands
(Rip - minutes to hours	blistering
	Burning or itching
	Dry skin
	Reaction limited to contact area
Allergic Contact Dermatitis (ACD)	*eczema
Type IV Hypersensitivity Reaction	severe itching
(Delayed - 6 to 48 hours)	vesicles/blisters
	Dryness
	Cracking
	Crusting
	Desquamation
	Reaction may extend beyond
	Glove area (up the arm)

*Appearance similar to irritant contact dermatitis; difference is the extent (within or Beyond glove border) of the reaction
*Chemical sensitivity falls within this type of reaction

Immediate Allergic Urticaria	itching
Type 1 Hypersensitivity Reaction	uricaria
(Immediate -minutes to 1 hour)	erythematic
	Edema
	Pruritis
	Swelling

TABLE IV. TRATING LATEX-ALLERGIC PATIENTS

• Identify the type of hypersensitivity reaction: (Type 1 or Type IV)

• Work closely with the patient's allergist

• Label the chart with an allergy alert sticker

• Schedule the patient early in the day (aeroallergens are at a minimum)

- Clear the counters, especially of any paper items

- Prepare the operatory with non-latex gloves

- If the room was disinfected using latex gloves, everything should be

- Wiped with water, including counters, bracket table, hand piece hoses,

- Chairs, x-rays, unit, and so forth

PAT FISH'S TATTOO SANTA BARBARA
Glove ALERT: ABOUT LATEX ALLERGY
Since Tattoo Artists have to use latex gloves, there is a potential threat for them the very item we now think of as standing as our first defense against cross-contamination with blood-borne diseases.

The Tattoo Artist worked his career for fifteen years ago. He learned the concept of sterile field, and he must maintain constant vigilance in their working environment. Mr. Cliff Raven was his Mentor and he was very aware of medical concepts, so therefore the latex glove has always been part of his Tattoo experience. It is important to not how recently they have become a part of tattooing, and how ubiquitous their presence is now.

After the tattoo artist wore the about five years, he noticed that he would break out in a rash. Especially when he wore the gloves for long periods, in the hot weather. He found out it was called contact dermatitis that is caused by direct contact with a substance. These little bumps were called comedomes, and by chance, if you scratch them they would become tiny open sores, perfect portals for entry of virus. When he learned that Vaseline commonly used to maintain the stencil on the skin is capable of braking down the latex, causing it to become porous (why they advise NOT to use petroleum products with latex condoms) He started changing them every twenty minutes and making sure that he let his hands cool off I between. He hears about latex allergy and causes were from the powder in the gloves. The powder acts as an abrasive substance, and wearing down the skin surface. The epidermal layer, which inviting the allergy-causing latex proteins to get into the body. He switched his gloves to non-powder-free latex. He stated that when he ate kiwi he coughed. The artist worked at the Mad Hatter's Tear Party in Portland Mine. This convention was very intense three-day event in room, artists and fans. He noticed that he had a weird barking cough.

He thought he had caught a virus or fungus on a plane ride. This cough continued and it seemed as though it could have been asthma, and he was running on reduced oxygen feeling like he was pre-pneumonial, and tired all the time. The artists decided to do some research on latex allergy because he wondered if he was sensitized. Since he had went to the convention most of the artist used powered latex gloves and that posed him over a toxicity limit and caused him to a toxicity limit and caused him to developed a greater sensitivity to latex. During his research, information scared him, it was a picture and article that who had the three-feet-across cloud of powder filling the air around it. One the powder is air-borne it can go into the lungs. Since we know now that the powder is a vehicle for transference for the proteins. The unpowdered gloves seemed to be safer because the process of making the gloves, these gloves go through chlorine wash the lower level of concentration so proteins on the surface by rising them away. Some people have problems wearing sneaker, or touch and ever a rubber band. In the home there are many thing made from-natural rubber latex. Fascinating substance whose discovery led to host of products making use of the unique qualities of this natural polymer, a chain of molecules that can be stretched out and then retain its shaper. Some people can no longer wear latex condoms. Which can be very serious? Working around latex once, you have been allergic to latex. There can be disastrous consequences, and latex-free living could get very confining. Even elastic is in underwear, pencil erasers, etc. For some people a little is too much. For me, I fell extremely lucky to have had the flash of inspiration to self-diagnose just in time, and that the cost of Nitrile gloves has dropped now to a manageable amount, not much more than latex. I consider it a small extra price to pay to continue in the occupation that I love. Since the last convention, he realized that it was in his best interest not to attend any more conventions to prevent allergic reactions. Much as I do not want to make myself into the poster child for this problem, informing my fellow tattoo artists of this very real threat to their continued ability to remain within this industry is very important to me. If this article saves, a few people some illness and allows them to continue their work. I've done my bit.

LETHAL LATEX

In the wake of the AIDS crisis, a number of health care worker have grown dangerously allergic to latex rubber. It almost cost this Arlington woman her life
By Carolyn Poirot, Writer for Star Telegram

Millicent Steffen, who is wearing latex-gloves, was diagnosed six weeks ago with latex allergy. When she has had episodes of anaphylactic reactions, similar to reactions to someone be allergic to bees. If Steffen comes in contact with latex she to administered epinephrine within one to two minutes and has 20 minutes to get to the hospital.

I'm going to die. I'm going to die, "Millicent Steffen sobbed over and over to the 911 emergency operator, gasping for breath and trying to convince her and husband, Keith, as he drove her to Arlington Memorial Hospital shortly after midnight on Nov. 6. She was covered with an itching red rash and she could not breathe. She did not want to take Ambulance because when was afraid it would kill her. Ambulances are full of latex, when would explain later, and it was the rubber that was causing her severe allergic reaction.

"It felt like I was smothering," Steffen recalled. "I couldn't breathe. It was as if I had peanut butter stock in my throat. My airway was totally shut down. I had hives all over from my head down. It was itching like I had ant bites everywhere.

Today, she calls it "the big one that almost killed me." Steffen, 31, was first treated for a severe allergic reaction Oct. 18 in the cardiac theorization lab at Columbia Medical Center of Arlington, where the worked as a radiology technician. Nobody guessed what caused the reaction, but the hives were obvious, and she was given an antihistamine and steroids by injection. When it happened again less than a week later, she was similarly treated in the hospital emergency room and referred in a specialist in immunology. A week later, she was waiting for the results of extensive blood tests when "the big one" hit. Like some other health care professionals throughout the country, she has developed a severe relation to latex, the natural sap of the rubber tree. Latex is used in an estimated 40,000 industrial products, including 400 routinely used in hospitals.

Steffen has worked in hospital - some days going through 30 or more pairs of latex gloves in a single eight-hour shift - for almost 10 years. She is now on medical leave, and coping with a life turned literally upside down. She must avoid exposure to latex in her personal life, as well no easy task considering that the rubber is used in such things as balloons, rubber-backed bathmats, cosmetic applicators, disposable diapers and many children's toys. She was given a list by her doctor to avoid is extensive.

She can't even take her kids to McDonald's any more because they often have balloons in there. She says. She had to throw always toys, because many had latex in them. Her husband opened up envelopes out side the house concern about the clue.

Last summer, the American College of Allergy, Asthma and Immunology warned that as many as 18 million Americans might be affected by latex sensitivity - 64 in every 1.000, up from 1 in 1,000 in the early 1980's. People, who work with medical supplies such as nurses and lab technicians, are particularly at risk for latex sensitivity because of their constant exposure to rubber, the ACAAI said. However, as the use of condoms and other consumer goods containing latex has risen, the general population has increasingly encountered latex products.

Warning on Hospital Gloves

Koop Criticized for Role in Warning on Hospital Gloves
By Holcomb B. Noble, The New York Times National
Friday, October 29, 1999

Dr. C. Everett Koop, who was Surgeon General in the 1980's. In the spring of 1997 Dr. C. Everett Koop, made a telephone call to Dr. Linda Rosen stock, director of the National Institute for Occupational Safety and Health. The Agency on way warn health workers that latex gloves widely used in hospitals could cause serious, even life-threatening allergic reactions. Dr. Koop told her the language of the warning was much overstated. Dr. Koop testified in the House on March 25 before the oversight and investigations subcommittee of the Work Force. Dr. Koop told the panel that the hazards being linked to the gloves by scientists and other health authorities were exaggerated. Borderline hysteria he called them. Mary Beith Zupa is a spokeswoman for Dr. Koop and she said that Dr. Koop had received substantial sums of money under a four-year, $1 million contract he signed in 1994 with a the leading manufacturer of the latex gloves, a relationship he did not disclose to Dr. Rosen stock or the subcommittee. Dr. Koop was not required to have registered as a paid lobbyist for the company since. He was not under contract with the glove manufacturer when he made the call to Dr. Rosenstock at NIOSH or testified before the subcommittee, which is headed by Representative Charlie Norwood, Republican of Georgia. Dr. Koop declined to discuss the matter. His has contacts with the glove maker WRP Corp. Did not last a full four years. NIOSH issued it warning anyway. Dr. Koop had an obligation to disclose his financial ties to NIOSH, in the Congress and the public. What this long admired and respected man has done in taking money from a glove manufacturer and then speaking out on its behalf is wrong, said Susan Wilburn senior specialist in occupational safety and health for the American Nurses Association. But worse, he has given very powerful help to an industry whose product is harming health workers and patients. Dr. Koop has long been one of the nation's most trusted health experts a reputation he gained as Surgeon General in the 1980's is battling the tobacco industry and focusing a reluctant nation on the seriousness of AIDS, among other efforts. Ms. Wilburn said an estimated 200,000 nurses had developed allergies and NIOSH studies show that 10 percent of health-care workers regularly exposed to the gloves and 17 percent with heavy exposure have developed allergies. More than 300 patients and workers file lawsuits. Some leading hospitals are Mayo Clinic, Johns Hopkins, have begun replacing powdered latex gloves with alternatives. Critics have found fault with steps that Dr. Koop and his business associates took to profit from his name and reputation, including establishing financial ties to companies whose products and services were described on a Web site he established. The critics say the glove contract is more troubling because it involves public policy and public health. According to filings with the Securities and Exchange Commission, the glove company contract called for Dr. Koop to deliver four speeches a year on health and nutrition. He was an advisor and gave the company the right to use his name, picture, speeches and biographical information. The contract also entitled Dr. Koop to a five-year option to buy 500,000 shares of company stock at 1994 prices, and a percentage of the net sales of nutrition products Ms. Supa said that Dr. Koop did not receive the full $1 Million called for in the contract; she would not say how much he received. There was a footnote to a WRP Corporation filing with the S.E.C. refers to an unmade individual who serves as a spokesman for the company and received $656,250 in consulting fees through Feb. 1997.

A representative of the company confirmed that the individual was Dr. Koop. Sanford Lewis, a lawyer for a group called Healthcare Without Harm formed to monitor health and safety in the medical field, said that Dr. Koop's activity on the glove issue and particularly his testimony in Congress had been influential. Would even Dr. Koop have sounded so convincing, Mr. Leis asked, if he had disclosed his financial deal with the glove company? Mr. Lewis said Dr. Koop's testimony in March was still being cited in state legislature as reasons to delay action on the gloves, even though it was based on a study that was never **done.** Dr. Koop had told Congress that he based his conclusions that concern about the gloves was unwarranted on a study by Centers for Disease Control. Nevertheless, the agency said later that it had not made such a study. The report Dr. Koop referred to was paid for, it turned out by another glove maker, Allegiance Healthcare Corporation, the author of the study said in a court deposition. Dr Koop said in an interview the he had been missed informed about the report's origin. Dr. Rosenstock of NIOSH said that Dr. Koop telephoned her as her agency was preparing its bulletin on the potential dangers of exposure to rubber latex gloves containing protein and powdered cornstarch. The powder is meant to make it easier to get the gloves off, but allergists say that when it mixes with the protein in the gloves t can cause severe allergic reactions leading on rare occasions to anaphylactic shock and five known cases, death, Dr. Rosenstock said. If the powder from the gloves is disbursed in the air, it can even affect people who have not worn the gloves. Dr Rosenstock, whose agency is a research division of the C.D.C. said Dr. Koop told her he had seen a draft of the NIOSH bulletin. She said his view was that it would cause more harm than good, because it might frighten hospital workers out of using gloves that protect them in handling infectious materials, Dr. Rosenstock said. I assured him that we had sent the bulletin out for peer review and I was confident that it was well based scientifically, she said, and in the end, the agency issued the bulletin including language in the final version that Dr. Koop objected to. The bulletin suggested that health workers use nonlatex gloves for activities not involving infectious materials and that if they choose latex gloves for handling infectious materials, and that if they chose latex gloves for handling infectious materials, they use the powder-free kind with reduced protein content. Since then, the Food and Drug Administration, the Occupational Safety and Health Administration and a number of scientists, including members of the American Academy of Allergies, Asthma and Immunology, all have taken the same basic position. Sheldon Krinshy, a professor in urban and environmental policy at Tufts University who has written extensively in science journals on disclosure issues, said of Koop's role in the glove issue, anyone who attempts in public forum to influence public policy has an absolute obligation to disclose any financial interests he has or has had within a time frame that could be perceived to represent a bias—and it certainly did in the Koop cases. Dr Sidney M. Wolfe, a physician and director of Public Citizen's Health Research Group, which sought unsuccessfully in 1988 to have the powdered-gloves banned from all hospitals, said. The whole issue with these gloves is a no brainier. Powdered gloves are causing serious problems. They're causing hospitals to lose workers who become disabled and there are perfectly good alternatives to that type of glove— and Dr. Koop has absolutely no scientific basis for the position he has taken. In response to criticism, an NIOSH spokeswoman said that the current warning seemed to sufficient but that the agency was considering whether to take active enforcement action.

Is occupational latex allergy causing your patient's asthma? Hives and "hay fever" symptoms are common warning signs. Journal of Respiratory Diseases, April 2002 B. Lauren Charous; Margaret A. Charous.

ABSTRACT: Given the prevalence of latex allergy in health care workers and others who wear latex gloves, it is prudent to maintain a high index of suspicion in patients with occupational exposure. In the US, confirmation of suspected latex allergy relies on serologic tests that are significantly less sensitive than skin prick test methods that are available in Canada and Europe. Specific inhalation challenge is the gold standard for the diagnosis of occupational asthma, but is not commonly available. In the 1999, more than 15 billion pairs of gloves were sold in the US. Hence, about 10 years ago, reports of anaphylactic reactions to latex (including some deaths) were surprising. Two distinct high-risk groups were initially identified: children with spinal bifida (although later it became apparent that any infant who underwent frequent surgical procedures was at risk) and patients who had undergone radiological examinations that used latex rubber barium enema retention balloons. Fortunately, institution of prophylactic safety measures has virtually eliminated serious reactions in these patients.

Although a topic persons are more likely to become allergic to latex than none a topic person, the key determinant of latex sensitization is exposure. Population prevalence studies that have used the skin prick test, the most accurate assessment tool, have reported positive test results in 5% to 12% of latex-exposed worker (5-7). Nearly half of these sensitized workers reported a history of allergic reactions.

In one study, 50% of allergic workers with no history of asthma experienced an asthmatic response during a "glove handling" inhalation challenge. (8) This suggests that long-term exposure to latex aerosol can provoke lower airway inflammatory responses and asthma. Observed rates of 2% to 10% for occupational asthma (OA) in workers who had long-term exposure justify concern. (7,9,10) However, only 2% to 3% of nonexposed a topic persons and only about 1% of the general population have positive skin test results. More, important, allergic symptoms are symptoms are rarely reported in these groups. (2,5,11)

Three of these studies examined the effects of latex exposure on "new job entrants," a group particularly relevant to understanding the nature of occupational risk.(12-15). Tarlo and colleagues (12) reviewed cross-sectional rates of latex sensitization and allergy in University of Toronto Dental School students and faculty none of the first- and second-year dental students who were tested were allergic. However, 5% of third-year and 10% of the fourth-year students had become sensitized. A quarter of faculty who were tested was allergic, and 10% had asthma (Figure).

Levy and associates (13) performed a similar study on dental students in London and Paris. None of 86 preclinical students had a positive skin test result. However, of the 189 graduating students, 11(6%) were allergic to latex.

An impressive prospective study of the University of Montreal and McGill University assessed the incidence of occupational allergy and asthma in more than 750 apprentice workers in 3 diverse categories: animal health technology, pantry-making, and dental hygiene technology. (14,15) On entry, the prevalence of latex allergy was insignificant in all 3 groups; however, during the course of the study, striking differences emerged.

Among the dental hygiene technology apprentices, who used latex gloves regularly, latex allergy became more widespread. Over 32 months, the cumulative incidence in the group for latex sensitization was 6.4% and for OA was 4.5% (15) Underlining the potency of latex as aeroallergen, the likelihood of latex sensitization in the dental hygiene technology apprentices was greater than the likelihood of latex sensitization in dental hygiene technology apprentices was greater than the likelihood of animal-derived allergen sensitization, in the animal health technology apprentices. (15)

Levy and colleagues (13) noted that latex allergy was not evenly distributed among the dental students but, rather, was confined to those who had used powered latex gloves. In fact, none of the 93 graduating dental students who had used only powder-free protein-poor gloves was allergic to latex.

Baur and associates (16) reported analogous findings in the study of airborne latex aero allergic exposure. They screened 145 persons and performed aeroallergen sampling in 32 hospital and operating rooms and physicians' offices. (16) Latex aeroallergen concentration varied widely, ranging from undetectable evidence of latex allergy; however, all o f the persons, who were sensitized, had worked in area where the aerosol concentration was at least 0.6 ng (m.sup.3). This suggests that, as with other industrial and indoor allergens, such as dust mites, a threshold for latex aeroallergen may be associated with the development of sensitization and subsequent symptoms.

Sources and routes of exposure:

Latex exposure takes place either through direct. One of the route are of exposure are the when you wear the latex gloves regularly, with some people with contact dermatitis. Which normal barrier function of the skin has been disturbed? Numerous aerosol-sampling studies have found appreciable levels of aeroallergen in medical settings, concentrations ranging less than 1 to more 300 ng/{m.sup.3}. When nonpowered latex or non-latex gloves are substituted for powdered latex gloves, latex aeroallergen levels predictably disappear, even when no other preventive measures are taken. In room without carpeting latex aerosol levels become undetectable within hours. (18,21) The initial aeroallergen sampling confirmed out suspicious that latex aerosol had dispersed into her work are (12 to 14 ng/ {m.sup.3} from other areas where powdered latex ng/ {m.sup.3} and in all other operatories, hygiene rooms, and laboratories sampled (14 to 90 ng/ng/{msup.3}. Substitute nonpowdered latex gloves throughout the office was effective in reducing concentration in the work area to below 5ng/{m.sup.3}. Multiple independent observations strongly suggest that implementation of appropriate glove procurement polices may eliminate latex aerosol and prevent both sensitization of glove wearers and inadvertent secondary exposure of patients with latex allergies.

Presentations of latex allergy

Some symptoms of latex allergy are uric aria, contact reactions or acute erythematic with purities, this can happen glove distribution. Acute dyshidrotic reaction can occur when is like protein contact dermatitis. The diagnosis of contact dermatitis is considered patients who rashes persist beyond several hours or that can be chronic. There are cases of patients had a nonspecific irritant dermatitis, also allergic contact sensitivity to rubber accelerators, as thiuram, are not infrequent, and patch testing can provide a definitive diagnosis. Latex allergy can cause a broad spectrum of respiratory complaints, in some cases there are patients that notice worsening symptoms since exposure at there work place. We believe that this is the cause of some patients with upper respiratory tract symptoms, such as sneezing, ocular, tearing an itching, severe rhino-rhea, and nasal stuffiness and may be indistinguishable from acute seasonal allergic rhinitis. Some patients are not aware of this and should be screened and tested. Some patients have lower respiratory tract complaints may range from a classic syndrome of wheezing and shortness of breath occurring or worsening at work to chronic cough. The course of OA is insidious. Asthma can gradually worsening or be missed or may not be recognized as result of exposure while at work. Latex allergic patient can have a chronic cough who has no evidence of air-way hyperactivity may be due to eosinophilic bronchitis.

Diagnostic considerations.

Assessment for possible latex allergy is mandatory before any medical, dental or surgical procedure that involves use of latex devices or gloves. If patients have a history of current or previous occupational latex, exposure and possible reactions should be sought. If there is any respiratory reaction that have been induced by any of theses listed below:

* An exposure to powdered latex gloves

* Severe allergies to foods know to cross-react with natural rubber latex, such as avocado,

Banana, kiwi, and hazelnut

* Introperative anaphylaxis

* Reactions caused by commercial latex products, such as condoms and balloons

Some patient have had hand eczema are so common among health care workers it can be dismissed, complaints occurred when wearing gloves. Contact dermatitis has been shown to be an independent risk factor fro development of latex allergy. That is why patients would be questioned about changes in nature of eczematous rashes-positive response may indicate the conversion from contact dermatitis to IgE-mediated allergic disease.

Evaluation of occupational latex allergy and asthma is hindered by FDA-approved shin test reagents. Some practitioners have used "homemade" glove extracts as reagents, because of the risk of systemic reactions; we recommend that this be done using only established protocols and appropriate reagent potency and stability testing with pooled anti-latex sera.

There is another approach uses any of FDA-cleared serologic assays for detection of anti-latex IgE. Unfortunately, these assays perform below the standards of skin prick test. Thus attempts is conform a "true" diagnosis in patient with convincing history of latex allergy may be confused by false-negative results.

Impact in the patient

Symptoms of frequent of acute attacks of severe asthma or anaphylaxis or pervasive sensations

Of shortness of breath, chest tightness, and difficulty in breathing may be hard to assess in some patients. Patient's complainants of acute or repeated attacks occurring in public place, shoe stores, libraries, restaurants, and gas stations, in absence of an identifiable source of latex exposure are not well explained as an allergic reaction to latex. Confusing symptoms and an absence of clearly defined triggers may tempt you to minimize the patient's distress or to attribute ambiguous symptoms to malingering. Malingering, however, is an uncommon diagnosis, particularly in persons who have had stable work histories and life situations and who have achieved professional accomplishments. More likely, the ubiquity of latex and the multiplicity of cross-reactive foods may create a state of hypervigilance.

Consider the possibility that previous "bona fide" acute reactions including anaphylaxis, may lead to a state that is characteristic of anxiety reactions (fight or flight response") It has been appreciated for some time that asthma provoked a high level of anxiety, and the symptom overlap between panic respiratory disease may confound diagnostic clarity.

Fear reactions resulting from suggestion, social contagion or experience with an aversive allergic event may prompt the patient to establish conditioned responses that eventually may lead to generalization to a whole class of similar stimuli, Conditioned fear responses that mimic latex allergy as pseudo allergic relations, may even intensify allergic and asthmatic reactions. The effects of these anticipatory attacks can be self-reinforcing and lead to social withdrawal, including agoraphobia in some severe cases. The decrements in quality of life and sense of well-being in such patients cannot be overstated.

Management

The cornerstone of successful management of occupational latex allergy and asthma is cessation of exposure. Since powdered latex gloves are the only significant source of workplace latex aeroallergen, workers who are not exposed to contaminated fluids, such as food handlers, should be provided exclusively with nonlatex gloves. Where latex gloves are used, only nonpowdered nonsterile gloves (examination gloves) should be used. Sterile latex gloves are an uncommon cause of problems in nonsensitized persons. For this reason, use of low-protein powdered surgical gloves (less than 50 {mu}g/g of ASTM D5712) instead of nonpowdered glove is acceptable if an ongoing assessment for the development of allergic reactions is maintained. Because the cost of conversion is not appreciable, the sales of nonpowdered latex examinations gloves have already surpassed the sales of powdered latex examination gloves. This appears to be the most likely explanation for precipitous decline in new patient's latex OA referrals seen at our center and reported by other tertiary referral institutions. The institution of appropriate glove precautions in the workplace has permitted the safe return to work of almost all of our latex-allergic employees.

Patients with hand dermatitis including contact dermatitis should be treated aggressively with both topical corticosteroids and moisturizers. You should be aware to be discouraging the use of petroleum-based skin moisturizing products under latex gloves. Which this compromises the barrier properties of latex rubber. If you notice continuing reactions while using latex gloves, it

Would be wise to change to nonlatex gloves. Workers with contact uric aria or symptoms of occupational allergic rhinitis who have confirmatory skin or serologic tests must avoid latex exposure. The routine use of {beta}-blockers by such patients is contraindicated, since these agents may block therapeutic response to drugs used for treatment of anaphylaxis. Patients with seasonal or perennial rhino conjunctivitis my benefit form intranasal corticosteroids. However, we ask patients to refrain from routine use of antihistamines so that the appearance of acute symptoms at work can be used as warning signal.

Treatment of OA follows the standard guidelines for nonoccupaitonal asthma. With persistent asthma symptoms, use of inhaled corticosteroids, sometimes at high doses or supplemented with an initial burst of oral corticosteroids, is required. The addition of other asthma therapy, including long-acting bronchodilators, leukotriene receptor antagonists, and theophylline, may be helpful and should be considered on patent-by patient basis. Since cough frequently accompanies latex OA, dry-powder inhalers are often better accepted by patients.

There are other contributing factors to asthma, sinusitis, gastroersophageal reflux disease, vocal cord dysfunction, as their allergic exposures, should be sought diligently ad treated. Despite aggressively treatment and cessation of exposure, asthma may persist for months or years after a patient has resigned from a job.

It is essential to appreciate the psychological impact of a diagnosis of latex, OA. Workers who are unable to maintain their current profession may have to cope with significant financial stresses and a threatened sense of self-esteem. For those whose primary identification is with their job (I'm an ICU nurse), the diagnosis of latex allergy can mean "the loss of life as you know it." Referral to a psychologist or mental health practitioner with expertise in treating persons with chronic illness and an understanding of latex allergy can help restore a patient's quality of life and promote a healthier adaptation to his or her circumstances.

Latex Allergy Among Emergency Workers
Merginet Medical Resource
By Aimee J. Frank

January 2004, Merginet - Latex allergies continue to plague emergency medical services, other healthcare professionals, and their patients. NIOSH official reported in April 2003 that an estimated eight percent to 12 percent of healthcare workers are latex sensitive, and Food and Drug Administration received more than 1,000 reports of latex-related health problems, in 15 deaths, between 1988 and 1992. The EMS workers are continuing using the gloves; they are particularly prone to the disorder because of repeated exposure to protective latex gloves. A 2001 study published in the American Journal of Epidemiology examined workers in occupations where latex gloves were latex gloves were used regularly to measure whether these workers displayed a greater sensitization to latex. The study found no greater prevalence to latex sensitization among healthcare workers. After controlling for the other factors associated with latex sensitization, the study authors said there was no significant association between longest-held jobs in healthcare and latex sensitization. The data for study were from the Third National Health and Nutrition Examination Survey (1988-1991) (NHANES 111) and included information from laboratory tests and surveys for 5,512 adults between 17and 60 years of age.

Allergy Testing

Warshaw notes that three types of tests can confirm a diagnosis of latex allergy: skin tests, inviro serologic tests and provocative tests. Most experts believe a skin prick test with diluted latex antigen is most sensitive, but it is unavailable in United States said Warshaw.

Latex-Free Options

Though medications may reduce allergy symptoms, the most effective way to avoid allergic reaction is to Avoid direct contact with product of natural rubber latex products, according the June 1997 NIOSH Alert "Preventing Allergic Reactions to Natural Rubber Latex in the Workplace.

Unfortunately, avoidance may be difficult due to the prevalence of medical items made with latex. Latex gloves are the most obvious problem, but the other equipment and supplies, such as adhesive bandages, oral and nasal airways, intravenous tubing, electrode pads, and stethoscopes and blood pressure cuffs, may also trigger reactions.

The good news is that as many facilities begin to maintain latex-free areas for their employee and patients, medical equipment manufacturers and suppliers have an increasing variety of latex-free products available to healthcare professionals. If you have reactions from latex, products please contact doctor for testing for latex allergy. Please wear medical alert bracelets so that the Medical Staff are aware of your medical condition.

Today's News

Despite Deaths, Study Shows EMTs Not Authorized to Administer Epinephrine in Most States Food Allergy & Anaphylaxis Network

Millions of Americans suffer from allergy to food, insect sting, latex, exercise, and medications. Many of these individuals are at risk for anaphylaxis, a potentially life-threatening allergic reaction. An estimated 84,000 anaphylactic episodes can be expected in the United States each year, resulting in as many as 550 deaths, according to a 1999 study.

Many who suspect the onset of an anaphylactic episode call 911 for emergency treatment. However, Emergency Medical Technicians (EMT's) responding to such a call may not be equipped with and authorized to administer epinephrine, a live-saving drug.

There are fatalities to anaphylaxis have resulted when there was delay in the administration of epinephrine, or epinephrine wasn't administered at all in a number of cases. The patient died en route to the emergency room, attended by EMTs who were not equipped with epinephrine.

There are tree categories that EMTs fall in: Baci, Intermediate, and Paramedic, with EMT-Basics by far the most numerous (comprising roughly 72% of all Mets nationwide.) Surprisingly, however, only twelve States currently authorize all EMT-Basic within their borders to carry and administer epinephrine. This means that individuals in thirty-nine States (including the District of-Columbia) experiencing an anaphylactic reaction run the risk of calling 911 and having EMT- Basic arrive at he scene unauthorized to carry and administer epinephrine.

Anne Munoz-Furliong is founder and CEO of the Food Allergy an Anaphylaxis Network (FAAN) states that It's really disconcerting that in a majority of States it's a roll of the dice whether the EMT who responds to the emergency call would actually have and be able to administer this life saving drug. FAAN and its members have spearheaded a national effort aimed at getting more States to implement laws or regulations authorizing all EMTs to be equipped with and authorized to administer epinephrine. .

.FAAN has recently released "Emergency Medical Services Epinephrine Policies, "a study that addresses the policies in force in each State regarding epinephrine and EMTs. A state-by-state EMT "report card" is posted on http://foodallergy.or/advocacy.html#emt. Members of the medical profession, the media, legislative staffers, Emergency Medial Service personnel, and concerned citizens may purchase a copy of the study by contacting the FAAN office 1-800-4040.

FAAN is a national nonprofit organization dedicated to increasing public awareness of, providing education about, and advancing scientific research on food allergies and anaphylaxis. Established in 1991, FAAN has over 23,000 members in the U.S., Canada and 62 other countries.

SOURCE Food Allergy & Anaphylaxis Network **Web Site:** http://www. foodallergy.org.

http://foodallergy.org/advocacy.html#emt

Emergency Medical Technicians (EMT's) and Epinephrine
The Food Allergy & Anaphylaxis Network

FAAN had learned that there are three types of EMT's: Basics, Intermediates, and the Paramedics in the 1998. There were only a small number of states would actually allowed all of its EMT's to have access to epinephrine and to administer epinephrine to a patient that was suffering from anaphylaxis. The vast majority of states only granted Paramedics (and sometimes Intermediates) this authorization. That was a surprise, because EMT's-Basics generally made up the majority of the EMT's in any given state. Basics, however, ere not permitted to even carry and administer epinephrine. Basics could only assist a patient in administering the patient' own prescribed epinephrine. The policy clearly overlooks the possibility that a patient, or patient's family, may not be in possession of prescribed epinephrine at the time of a reaction if occurred. Since this discovery, FAAN members, along with medical professionals, allergists, lawmakers, and emergency personnel undertook an initiative to implement laws or regulations that would make the epinephrine more available from EMT-Basic in all states. The laws or regulations have been enacted in 26 states over the last five years: New York and Washington (1999); Connecticut (2000); Colorado, Iowa, Illinois, Louisiana, and Texas (2001); Indiana, Kansas, Kentucky, Massachusetts, Maryland, Maine, Minnesota, Mississippi, New Hampshire and Oklahoma (2002); Idaho, Michigan, Missouri, Nebraska, New Jersey, North Carolina and Pennsylvania (2003); Virginia (2004); and Arizona (2005).

NEW LEGISLATION IN WASHINGTON, DC

Jim Graham a DC Council Member has introduced the Emergency Access to Epinephrine Act of 2005. This bill states that all EMT's in the District to be trained to use the epinephrine auto-injectors, and requires that the devices to be kept on board all licensed ambulances. This bill protects EMT's from civil liability in the event that they administer an epinephrine auto-injector in conformity with appropriate emergency medical protocol.

NEW REGULATIONS IN ARIZONA

Earlier this year, the Arizona Bureau of EMS adopted new regulation that will allow EMT-Basic in the state to access and administer epinephrine auto-injectors. Due to the parents in Arizona these new regulations are largely do to them. Their voices supported for the change.

THE NATIONAL MAP

As a result of recent developments (such as the new regulations in (Arizona), FAAN has reconfigured the national map regarding EMT's and epinephrine. Each state (including the District of Columbia) has been place into one of three categories according to its EMT's epinephrine policy. This classification, though based on correspondence between FAAN and state EMS agencies, should not be considered absolutely precise, because decisions pertaining to EMT"s often vary within each state. FAAN has always advised that individuals contact their state EMS agency and their local ambulance provider in order to clarify the coverage in their particular locality.

GROUP A (EXCELLENT COVERAGE)

All EMT's are authorized, by law or regulations, to access, and administer epinephrine:

Connecticut	**New Hampshire**
Florida	**North Carolina**
Illinois	**Oregon**
Kentucky	**Rhode Island**
Louisiana	**Tennessee**
Massachusetts	**Washington**
Maryland	**Wisconsin**
Michigan	**Wyoming**
Minnesota	

Total: 17

GROUP B (LOCALITY-DEPENDENT)

The legal/regulatory framework is in place that allows all EMT's to access and administer epinephrine, but this is determined by local factors such as optional training and /or local medical control. In the case of Delaware, and Hawaii, EMT-Basics are not allowed to access and administer epinephrine;

however, due to small size of the states, Advanced Life Support (ALS) ambulances staffed by Paramedics cover virtually the entire area.

Alaska
Arizona
California
Colorado
Delaware
Georgia
Hawaii
Idaho
Indiana
Iowa
Kansas
Maine
Mississippi
Missouri

Nebraska
New Jersey
New Mexico
New York
North Dakota
Ohio
Oklahoma
Pennsylvania
Texas
Virginia
Washington, DC

Total: 25

GROUP C [NEEDS IMPROVEMENT]

EMT-Basics are not allowed to access and administer epinephrine, and may only assist a patient in administering the patient's own prescribed epinephrine auto-injector.

Alabama
Arkansas
Montana
Nevada
South Carolina

South Dakota
Utah
Vermont
West Virginia*

Total: 9

New protocols have received preliminary acceptance, and should advance West Virginia into Group B during the coming months.

FAAN hopes that soon EMT/epinephrine coverage will be seamless across the nation, so that no matter where an individual experiences and anaphylactic episodes, EMT's will arrive at the scene both equipped with epinephrine, and authorized to administer this precious medication.

If you're interested in helping improve the state affairs regarding EMT's and epinephrine in your state, please email **Christopher Weiss**, FAAN's Director of Legislative and Regulatory Research. The Food Allergy & Anaphylaxis Network (1-800-929-4040

Latex Allergy Guidance

Wednesday 15ᵗʰ September 2004
By Smile-on.com.
The future of density is here

The Faculty of General Dental Practitioners [FGDP] UK is launching the latest in their Good Practice Guidelines series: Guidance for the management of Natural Rubber Latex allergy in dental patients and dental healthcare workers.

There is a need to correct the protocols to protect individuals from latex sensitivity. There have been increasing incidents. This issue is very important and recently brought into focus the award of significant damages to a nurse. In Wales, who suffered allergic reactions to latex gloves, while she was working in the hospital in the 1980's and 90's.The publication consists of practical, evidence-based tips and details the importance of setting up and adhering to policies for the prevention and management of natural rubber latex allergy (NRL). The document gives guidance on the need to educate workers, and patients, as well as protocols for referral the experts for investigation and management of individuals with symptoms of allergy. It also suggests when NRL gloves should be used gloves should be used and the type of gloves of choice powder free and low protein.

Following is a summary of the important point to remember:

Dentists must have policies for the prevention of management of NRL allergy
All dental HCWs (healthcare workers) must be educated about the recognition and management of NRL allergy for both patients and

themselves. Immediate referral for specialist investigation and management should be instigated for patients and dental HCWs who develop signs and symptoms suggestive of
type 1 allergy to NRL.

- NRL gloves should only be used where there is an operational need.

- If NRL gloves are worn they must be powder free and low in protein.

The new guidance will be launched at 12pm on 15 October 2004 at the FGDP (UK) stand (B02) at the London Dental Showcase.

Previous publications in the PGDP(UK) Good Practice Guidelines series are Selection Criteria for Dental Radiography. Clinical Examination and Record Keeping and Antimicrobial Prescribing in Primary Dental Care for General Dental Practitioners.

There is also a new edition of Selection Criteria for Dental Radiography, which has been fully revised by a team of experts. Several sections have been updated in the light of new evidence and research finding while others, such as the use of digital radiography, have been expanded to reflect an increasing use in general dental practice. These selection criteria also conform to the Ionising Radiation (Medical Exposure). Regulations (IRMER) Implemental in 2000, and will help practitioners form a sound basis for clinical decisions.

PALATIN FIRE DEPARTMENT
Monthly Report February 2004

PFD Ambulances outfitted with Latex Free equipment

Throughout February, the EMS department had been busy retrofitting, all current
EMS's equipment to "latex-free" products. Considering the increasing number of citizens, as well as many healthcare personnel, who have developed sensitivity to all varieties of latex products, Northwest Community Hospital has instituted measures to accommodate this up and coming problem. So, as of February, all EMS's providers in the NWCH EMS System had to comply their ambulances and EMS equipment to latex-free

STANDARD OPERATING GUIDELINESDELTA CARDIFF
VOLUNTERR
FIRE COMPANY

S.O.G E57-Revision 0

SUBECT:Latex Allergies

DIVISION:Ambulance

INITIAL DATE: 26 June 2003EFFECTIVE DATE: 23 February 2004

PURPOSE: To provide guidelines to ensure safe care of the latex allergic patient and to prevent latex sensitivity allergic reactions among pre-hospital providers.

APPLICABLE TO: ALL EMS, Fire and Fire Police Members

AUTHORITY: DCYFC Ambulance Committee

Background

1.Latex is a common component of man medical products and has been found to cause severe allergic reactions. An allergic reaction to latex can occur with any contact between a latex product and the skin. More severe reactions have been seen with parental or mucous membrane contact and with inhalation latex particle. Symptoms can appear with 10 minutes but can take up to two hours to appear. Reactions may include hives, skin rashes, swelling, itching, runny eyes, nasal congestion, shortness of breath, wheezing, abdominal cramps, diarrhea, anaphylactic shock, and death.

2. Latex allergic individual are those who have experience systemic anaphylactic symptoms such as Itching swelling, hives, or difficulty breathing after exposure to various

Latex products or foods such as, bananas, chestnuts, and avocados.

3. Latex sensitive individuals are those who have only experienced local skin reaction only and may be in a high risk group (see below) or sensitive to such foods describe above

4. Patients with high risk for developing a latex allergy include:

A. Patients with a history of Spina Bifida, bladder Exstrophy, and congenital Urological Abnormalitites

B. Patients with a history of multiple allergies or allergies to nuts

C. Patients with a history of allergic reactions after touching balloons, rubber gloves (or powder in them), or consumer latex products.

D. Patients who have an unexplained anaphylactic reaction during surgery, at the dentist or during urinary catheterization or other bladder/vaginal /rectal stimulation.

Guidelines

1. Non-latex gloves shall be standard stock. Every attempt shall be made to supply non-latex products and equipment.

2. All patients should be asked allergy status and that reported to the next caregiver.

3. If the patient is latex allergic or sensitive, patient contact with any latex products shall be avoided during care. If a latex-containing product must be used (i.e., blood pressure cuff), a barrier shall be used between the item and the patient's skin. A 0.22 micron filter should be used, if available, to administer intravenous medications (especially those drawn up through a latex stopper or run through a latex port).

4. If the patient develops a latex allergic reaction during transport, he/she shall be treated as per appropriate medical protocols. Any reactions shall be reported to the next caregiver and documented on the Patient Care Report.

5. If a crewmember is latex allergic or develops latex sensitivity, he/she shall notify an EMS officer, in order that all precautions may he taken to minimize exposure.

6. It is highly recommended that the crewmember have proper allergic identification and he treated by a physician for the latex allergy/sensitivity.

Approved: /s/ Anthony Hall

Title: Vice President

Latex nipple.
(On formula bottles could caused infant allergy)
Pediatrics for Parents, April 2002 v20i4p2(1)

Latex allergies are somewhat rare in children. They usually occur in children who have had many exposures to latex-containing medical devices. Most of these children suffer from congenital defects of the spine (neural tube defects) or chronic genitourinary problems.

A recent case reminds us that children with no known history of such latex exposure may have a latex allergy. In this case, a two-month-old bottle-fed infant was brought to the emergency room because of strider (an abnormal, high-pitched, musical breathing sound caused by a partial blockage in the throat or larynx). The infant had a history of eczema. He was on a soy-based formula as it was thought he was allergic to cow's milk.

It turned out the problem wasn't the formula but the nipple. Many bottle nipples contain latex. One the baby was switched to a latex-free, silicon nipple the episodes of stridor disappeared.

Annals of Emergency Medicine 4/02.
This database brought to you by, Heath Reference Center Academic
http://web7.infotrac.galegroup.com/itw/informark/149/832/42672506w7/pul=rcl_HRCA-

Lip, Swollen
(Allergic Reaction). B.D. Schmitt
Clinical Reference System, Annual 2001 p1202

Description
The sudden swelling of a lip that hasn't been injured is usually caused by an allergic reaction to something that has gotten n the lip. If it is an allergic reaction, a child will also have symptoms of itching or tingling

Causes
The substance causing the reaction can be a food, toothpaste, lipstick, or lip balm. Other irritants (for example, an evergreen resin) may be on the lip from the hands.

Home Care (for local allergic reactions)
Wash the lips and face with soap and water to remove any irritating substance (decontamination)

Apply ice to the swelling for 20 minutes out of every hour. This should reduce the swelling and the itch. Repeat this for 3 hours if necessary.

Give an antihistamine in the correct dosage. (Benadryl is best) Continue 2 or 3 times. If Benadryl is not available, use any over-the counter hay fever or cold medicine.

Avoid any allergic foods that are associated with the lip swelling.

Please inform your Child's Physician Immediately if allergic reactions persist.

Marion Ronee Daney

Oregon soon to ban latex glove use:
Foodservice workers will not be allowed
To use latex rubber gloves beginning in
Scott Human. Restaurants & Institutions, Oct 15, 2002 v112 i23
p.78 (1)

March 2003. (Small is Beautiful)

On March 1, 2003, Oregon joins a handle of other states that have prohibited use of latex in foodservices facilities. Studies have identified latex as an allergen for a small percentage of the population. The possible that allergens can be transferred from gloves to food also is a common. Changes had to be made effective in Jan 1, 2001, revisiting state food code, including recognizing HACCP principles as the basis for food-protection programs. There was a shift in glove use and some delayed to give foodservices operation additional time deleted glove inventories, and retrain staff.

Mr. Bill Perry, director of government relations for the organization, which argued that restaurateurs voluntarily could eliminate latex-gloves use where allergy concerns exist He also stated that "We aren't convinced the legislation is necessary Oregon Restaurant Association ORA), lobbed against the prohibition this new law does not cover healthcare workers. Occupational Health & Safety Administration estimations, that 8% to 12% of workers in professional are latex-sensitive. "We didn't agree with the ban, but we have worked with Oregon Department of Human Services all along, advising operation to provide alternatives gloves, says Perry's, and we will continue to do so. Our role is to educate our members about the new law and ways to live with it. ODHS estimates that half of all foodservice facilities use latex rubber gloves. For those that do the legislation will require some retraining, says Perrys. The form-fitting gloves, including those made from latex often are preferred according to ORA's feedback, but "they will simply have to adjust" to using single-use gloves in the coming months. Differences in state regulations concerning latex glove cause make it difficult for multistage chain operations in develop a single standard for their systems.

The 2001 Food and Drug Distraction Food Code prohibit foodservice employees from bare-handed contact with ready-to-eat foods, mandating that "deli tissue, spatulas, tongs, single-use gloves or dispensing equipment" be used. For food that is not ready to eat, the requirements are that bare-hand contact be minimized. The code's only prohibition related to use of cloth gloves for food handlers. Arizona and Rhode Island are among states that have legislated bans on latex gloves in foodservices. Massachusetts Department of Public Health and Wisconsin's Department of Health and Family Services have followed the National Institution of Occupational Safety and Health's lead in recommending-but not requiring-that latex gloves not to be used in foodservice.

LATEX ALLERGENS

{English | Japanese}

Latex allergens that have already been registered by <u>WHO-OUIS</u> can be tabulated with their predicted physiological roles as follows.

Table. Registered Natural Rubber-Latex Allergens

Name	Trivial name	Predicted physiological roles	References
Hev b 1	rubber elongation factor	rubber biosynthesis	1,2
Hev b 2	beta-1, 3-glucanases	defense-related protein	3,4
Hev b 3	small rubber-particle protein	rubber biosynthesis	2,5,16,17
Hev b 4	microhelix component	defense-related protein	3
Hev b 5	acidic latex protein	7	6,7
Hev b 6.01	prohevin, hevein preprotein		
Hev b 6.02	hevein	Defense-related protein	
Hev b 6.03	prohevein C-terminal domain	(latex coagulation)	4,8,9
Hev b 7	patatin-like proteins	inhibitor of rubber biosynthesis	10,11,12
(Hev b 7b)	Inhibitor of rubber biosynthesis (Hev b 7 c)		
Hev b 8	Latex profiling	structural protein	13,14,15
Hev.b 9	latex enolase	?	18
Hev b 10	Mn-superoxide dismutase	?	19
Hev b 11w	class 1 endochitinase	defense-related protein	20
Hev b 12	lipid transfer protein	defense-refense-protein	-

Official allergen list by WHO-OUIS
Allergen nomenclature
Allergen sequence database (BISF)
Monthly journal indexing on allergens and related articles (ISFA)
NIHS/DMD/yagam@nihs.go.jp
http://dmd.nihs.go.ap/latex/allergen-e.html

Rotavirus Infection in Children with Acute Diarrhea as detected by Latex Agglutination, ELISA and Polyacrylamide Gel Electrophoresis.

Authors: Altindis M: Yavrou SL Simsek A; Ozkul A: Ceri A: Koc H
Affiliation: Kocatepe University School of medicine, Department of Microbiology and Clinic Microbiology, Afyon, Turkey

Indian Pediatr (Indian pediatrics.) 2004 Jun; 41(6): 590-4

We examined prospectively, stool specimens from 135 children, 0 to 3 years old, referred for fever, abdominal pain, vomiting, and /or acute diarrhea. Rotavirus antigens were detected from facial samples by latex agglutination (LA), ELISA AND PLYACRYLAMIDE GEL ELECTROPHORESIS (page). Rotavirus antigen posterity by Latex, ELISA and PAGE were 15, 55%, 12.59% and 11.85%, respectively. With PAGE test as reference, the sensitivity and specificity of LA and ELISA tests was 93.75%, 94.96% and 100%, 99.16%, respectively, The positively ratio between 13-24 months group was meaningful with all tests (P = 0.042 for LA; P = 0.05 for ELISA; P – 0.031 for PAGE). ELISA and LA use found to be as sensitive and specific as PAGE in the diagnosis of rotavirus diarrhea.

Increased prevalence of latex-sensitization among children with chronic renal failure.

Authors: Dehlink E; Prandstetter C; Eiweggrt T; Urbanek R; Szepfalusi Z,
Affiliation: Department of Pediatrics, Division of General Pediatrics, Medical University of Vienna, Vienna, Austria

BACKGROUND: Type 1-allergy to natural rubber latex (NRL) has been shown to be more prevalent among certain groups of patients. Children suffering from chronic renal failure (CRF) could be a suspected risk group because of their intense exposure to latex through catheters, gloves and anesthetic equipment during frequent hospitalizations from early life on. We investigated the prevalence of latex-sensitization among this group of patients and sought to identify risk factors. METHODS; Ninety-three patient (mean age 10.5 years) suffering from CRF were assessed by questionnaire-based his to history (details on renal disease, number and kind of surgical procedures, family and personal history of atopic diseases, allergic reaction to NRL, and the use of pacifiers) and by measurement of total and latex-specific serum immunoglobulin (Ig) E. RESULTS: Ten of 93 (10.8) patients showed elevated latex-specific IgE-levels. One of 10 patients reported clinical symptoms to latex-allergen, but no allergic reactions to NRL during medical care were reported, Sensitized patients were significantly more likely to be atopic, reflected by a positive history of other allergies as well as elevated total serum IgE-levels, and had a significantly higher number of urogenital surgeries (P = 0.02 in all cases, Fisher's exact and Wilcoxon test, respectively). CONCLUSION: This study demonstrates that children with CRF are at increased risk of latex-hypersensitivity. Significant associations with atopy and repeated surgeries were observed. Large studies are required to elucidate whether these children are also at increased risk of anaphylaxis and therefore deserve preventive measures.

C. A. Reject Manufacturing-Defect Finding in First Latex Glove Trial

Fourth District Panel Says It Was Reasonable for Maker to Weigh One Safety Consideration Against Another Metropolitan News-Enterprise: By Kenneth Ofgang, Staff Writer/Appellate Courts: Friday 21, 2002

Evidence that a leading manufacturer of health care products could have done a better job of washing latex gloves, and this reduced protein levels that have been linked to serious allergies suffered by thousands of workers in hospitals and medical offices, did not prove that the gloves were defectively manufactured the Fourth District Court of Appeal ruled yesterday.

Div. One affirmed an order by San Diego Superior Court Judge William C. Pate, throwing out a jury verdict for close to $900,000 in the first latex glove product liability cast to go to trial in California. Pate has been assigned by Chief Justice Ronald M George as coordination judge to oversee more than 40 such cases from around the state.

There are several hundred cases pending throughout the United States, about two-thirds of them in federal courts and the rest in the courts of over 30 states.

Judgment NOV

The jurist granted The Manufacture Company's motion for judgment NOV in a suit brought by Christine McGinnis, a Stockton respiratory therapist whose doctors said she had contracted a life-threatening alley form wearing natural rubber latex gloves.

The Manufacture Company is a major supplier of hospital medical products, and sold 50 percent of the natural rubber latex gloves used in the United Stated before spinning off the unit that made the gloves.

McGinnis, who wore 30 to 50 pairs of gloves per day, said she experienced a severe allergic reaction in November 1995, while wearing gloves and was hospitalized in intensive care for six days. She later experienced over 35 allergic reactions to natural rubber products and had to quit work, she said

Experts' Claim

Plaintiffs' experts claim that 950,000 health care workers have been or may become sensitive to latex as a result of exposure to the protein in gloves. The allergic reaction has been said to range forma localized rash to systemic conditions such as hives, shortness of breath an life threatening anaphylactic shock, and the experts claim that simple 30-second process of washing the latex out of the gloves was known to industry bun not utilized by The Manufacture Company until 1996.

However, Justice Richard Huffman, writing yesterday for the appellate panel said the court counts not, as a matter pf pubic policy, holds that The Manufacture Company failure to use the washing process rendered the gloves defective.

The Manufacture Company presented evidence that these steps might lead to defects in barrier protections such as pinholes, tearing or a changing texture," the just explained. It was entirely reasonable, Huffman said, for The Manufacture Company to consider barrier protection issues before changing it manufacturing process.

Huffman also noted that the Food and Drug Administration did not require labeling of latex gloves for latex content untill1993 after The Manufacture Company had begun labeling them voluntarily and, that prior to 1998, the agency did not allow manufacturers to make comparisons of protein levels and had not adopted standards.

Efforts Ineffective

"We believe that Plaintiff's efforts are ineffective to show that the various... gloves that were manufactured precisely as intended that complied with applicable governmental standards, and that fulfilled their primary barrier function, never the less have manufacturing defects... reflective of the state of scientific knowledge regarding latex protein levels of exposure available to the relevant participants in this health care product context." The justice wrote

The case is *In re Coordinated Latex Glove Litigation*, 02 S.OS.3105.

In vivo and vitro in diagnosis of latex allergy at Groote Schuur Hospital
Department of Immunology, Groove Schuur Hospital, Cape Town
Authors: Marais GI; Fletcher JM; Potter PC

The aim of this study was to evaluate the diagnostic utility of skin-prick tests, radio-allergosorbent tests (CAP RASTs), basophile histamine release sulphidoleukotriene release and Western blotting in the diagnosis of latex allergy at Groote Schuur Hospital. DESIGN: Patients with a history suggesting latex hypersensitivity were recruited via staff health and allergy clinics at Groote Schuur Hospital. Clinical assessment by Laboratory investigation and skin-prick testing. The controlled group consisted of Laboratory and hospital staff that had regular latex exposure but were a symptomatic, SETTING: Hospital-based cohort at Groot Schuur Hospital. PARTICIPANTS: Twenty-three patients with suspected latex allergy; 10-control subjects exposed to, but not clinically sensitive to, latex. MAIN OUTCOME: Skin-pick testing was more sensitive than invitro diagnostic tests for the diagnosis of latex allergy. RESULTS: Eighteen of 21 (85.7%) of the patients tested had positive skin-prick test with commercial latex solution (Allerbioprick) and 17/21 (80%) tested skin-prick-positive with an in-house glove extract. CAP RASTs were positive in 13/23 patients (56.5%), sulphidoleukotriene release was positive in 10/23 (43%), histamine release assay was positive in 10/23 (45%) and Western blots were positive in 8/23 (34.7%). All patients with only urticaria were Western blot-negative and CAP RAST-negative, suggesting that they have very little circulating latex-specific IgE although patients who were Western blot-positive tended to have multi-organ involvement, both patients with anaphylaxis wee Western Blot-negative.

Conclusion: Latex allergy is a significant clinical problem at Groote Schuur Hospital. Titrated shin-prick testing performed in a controlled environment can safely and reliably confirm the diagnosis in patients who do not give a history of anaphylaxis. The CAP RAST was the most sensitive in vitro test for latex allergy locally available, but lacks sensitivity in patients presenting with urticaria only.

Chemical Susst: Leukotrienes {0}
Sulfhydryl Compounds {0}
Rubber {9006-04-6}
Descriptor: (Minor): Adult

CONDOM INFORMATION

HOW LATEX CONDOMS ARE MADE & TESTED

It takes a lot of work to make a condom that can stand up to the height of your passion! The makers of Durex condoms will take you behind the scenes to show you just what it takes to make some of the world's favorite condoms

The condoms by Durex are made from the finest quality natural latex. However, before the latex even reaches the manufacturing plant, it undergoes comprehensive quality control tests to ensure that it conforms to Durex's stringent specifications.

Once the latex passes quality control tests, it is processed into a useable form. Because latex is a natural material (very similar to milk in many of its physical properties), it can curdle or go sour. Stabilizers, preservatives and vulcanizing agents are added and the latex is checked again for the quality and consistency. This process is known as "compounding".

The next stage in manufacture is "dipping', the compound latex is fed into temperature controlled tanks into which a continuous line of glass formers are dipped. As the formers pass gently through the tanks they pick up an almost invisible layer of latex film. The latex coating is then dried using filtered air to prevent atmospheric contamination. After drying, the formers are dipped once more and dried again.

On completion of the dipping process, the open ends of the newly formed condoms are rolled to form a rim or bead. The condoms, while still on the formers, are then passed through an oven to vulcanize the latex. Before the condoms are removed form the formers by high-pressure jets of water, they undergo a soaking process to loosen the condoms from the former. They are dried.

Although Durex condoms are now ready for packaging, they will not reach that stage until they have undergone a series of 5 stringent tests. This adherence to high quality standards has made Durex the leading condom brand in the world today. With a product such as a condom, where quality is vitally important to the user. It is essential that every effort be made to ensure the perfection and reliability of every single one.

As well as the tests specified by national and international standards. Durex condoms are electronically tested. The in involves each condom being stretched over a metal former and subjected to a high voltage. Any breakdown of the film is measured and any minor flaw, even one far too small to be detected by the human eye, results in the condom being instantly rejected.

Perhaps the most impressive test is Air Inflation Test. This is carried out each and every day on samples of each batch of Durex condoms. This is the test of elasticity and strength that involves a Durex condom being filled with air until it reaches bursting point. Typically, a Durex condom holds approximately 40 liters of air, which is equivalent to 9 gallons of water, before bursting

Once electronic testing is complete, Quality Control samples are taken from each batch filled with 300ml of water, and suspended for 3 minutes. Afterwards they are examined for minute fluid leakage by rolling them on blotting paper. If more than small number displaying flaws are found, then the entire batch is rejected and scrapped.

Additional samples are checked for size and thickness. Further samples are tested to destruction for physical strength. Some of these samples are artificially aged at accelerated temperatures, as an assurance of their quality at the end of their 5-year product life.

This is where Justrubbers come in. We use a JIT (Just In Time) inventory system and buy directly from the manufacturers – not from us are the newest most reliable and current products available on the market today. There are many different kinds of condoms: Atlas, Beyond Seven, Durex, Female Condom, InSpiral, Kameleon, Kimono, LifeStyles, MAXX, Naturalamb, etc...

This above article was adapted from Durex Consumer Products. Visit their website at

ATTORNEY GENERAL WANT TO BAN LATEX GLOVES IN RHODE ISLAND FOOD INDUSTRY

PROVIDENCE BUSINESS NEWS

Providence—attorney General Sheldon Whitehouse has submitted legislation to General Assembly that would prohibit food businesses from using latex gloves.

According to the Attorney General's to Attorney General's office, the Latex Gloves Safety Act would ban any person, firm or corporation that operates a food business from using disposable, nonsterile and sterile latex gloves. The bill would also require non-food businesses using latex gloves to post a clear warning of the health risks of latex gloves.

A long with increase in latex use, the number of people with an allergy to the natural rubber has dramatically risen. The Food and Drug Administration reports that between January 1985 and March 1999, there were five deaths from allergies to latex gloves and 2,330 allergic reactions.

"Unfortunately, we see a significant increase (of allergic reactions) because of the increased use of latex gloves," said Jim Brady, a disability lawyer. Brady has represented more nurses with latex allergies than any other lawyer in New England. "I think, among many people, there's no awareness of the problem with latex gloves."

An allergic response generally triggers a poison ivy like rash 12 to 36 hours after contact. While this is not life threatening, some people may have a reaction to the latex protein itself. A full-blown allergic response often affects the skin and other organs, producing hives, swelling, asthma and, in extreme cases, anaphylactic shock.

Pandolfo has had reaction to food prepared by people wearing latex gloves, latex powder residue left on a table at the doctor's office, and, once, to a water glass that was handled by a girl wearing the gloves.

"I don't go out to eat any where unless I've talked to the chef first, "Pandolfo said, "This is life-threatening."

When she travels, she telephones the hotel ahead of time to talk with the chef. She brings her own food on an airplane. In addition, she only uses self-adhesive stamps.

"I can't lick a stamp. I can't lick an envelope, "she said. "(Latex) is out there everywhere, and you can just die."

While many hospitals have voluntarily changed to non-latex products, some health care facilities have been reluctant to discontinue its use. A majority of restaurants, day-care centers and beauty salons continue to use latex, unaware that they are messing with a deadly allergen.

"For the places that haven't changed over, education hasn't gotten out to the degree that it needs to," said Gail Lenehen, editor for the Journal of the Emergency Nurses Association. Lenehen went into anaphylactic shock three years ago while working in the emergency room of Massachusetts General Hospital in Boston. "They haven't reached the average nurse, physician or hairstylist.

In 1997, the National Institute of Occupational Safety and Health recommended that non-latex gloves be used for all activities that are not likely to involve contact with infectious materials, such as food preparation, routine housekeeping and maintenance. The same year, the Food and Drug Administration established rules for labeling all medical devices that contain latex.

While there are a number of non-latex products available, including gloves made of vinyl or polyvinyl chloride, nitrile or other synthetics, many hospitals are slow to change because of the additional cost.

"It's money," Brady said. "The vinyl gloves are not as cheap as latex gloves. The latex gloves are very accessible, very easy."

Brady said, however, that the health-case industry is under the false impression that latex gloves are always less expensive. He said a growing number of non-latex gloves are just as good `and priced competitively with latex.

"The pro-active actions that need to be taken, which are to eliminate latex gloves, are very doable, but there is tremendous reluctance at the facilities, said Evelyn Bain, associate director of occupational at the facilities, "said

Evenlyn Bain, associate director of occupational safety and health for the Massachusetts Nurses Association. "It doesn't make sense not to do it."

LATEX PAINT DOES NOT POSE A THREAT TO THOSE WHO
SUFFER FROM LATEX ALLERGIES

Public Affairs Division
National Paint & Coating Association

The National Paint & Coatings Association (NPCA) would like consumers to know that the type of latex found in latex paints is not the same type of latex found in products the trigger latex allergies. In s recent report aired on ABC television's "20/20" on March 14, 1997 – it was noted that commonly – used

Products containing latex have caused allergic reaction – sometimes severe –in approximately one to six percent of the population. These allergic reactions have most commonly been associated with surgical gloves and other natural latex products worn close to the skin.

The key distinction for latex in paint is that it is generally synthetic (polymerized from various monomeric materials, principally vinyl acetate and various acrylates) and dispersed in water. By contrast, the latex used in other products is usually naturally derived form rubber tree sap and contains, among other, hydrocarbon polymers and proteins. In particular, the protein component of natural latex is regarded as the likely cause of allergic reactions.

Because of these and other differences, consumers need not be concerned about using latex paint and developing the allergic reactions that have been associated with natural latex.

ARE LATEX AND FOOD ALLEGIES RELATED?

Recently, coincident IGE- medicated allergies to latex and multiple fruits or vegetables have been documented. In *vivo and in vitro* investigations of clinical specificity have produced complex patterns of allergenic cross-reactivity (suggesting shard or common antigenic components) among botanically uncrated allergens such as latex ad food. While the details of the clinical relationship between latex and food allergies await further study, documentation of food allergies known to coexist with latex sensitivities may be useful for identifying the risks of latex exposure for some patients

Listed below; are the allergens reported to be associated (clinically or immunochemically) with natural rubber latex.

Degree of Association or Prevalence

High	Modern	Low	or undetermined
Banana	Apple	Pear	Rye
Avocado	Carrot	Peach	Wheat
Chestnut	Papaya	Cherry	Grass
	Kiwi	Pineapple	Ragweed
	Tomato	Strawberry	Mugwort
	Potato	Fig	Hazelnut
	Melon	Grape	Walnut
		Apricot	Soybean
		Passion Fruit	Peanut
		Plums	Nectarine
		Mango	

`Simultaneous occurrence of allergies to certain pollens and foods described above have also been documented in reports independent to those focusing on natural rubber latex. Significant levels of allergenic cross-reactivity have been demonstrated for the allergen groups listed below:

Mugwort with carrot, celery, apple, peanut and kiwi

Birch with apple, pear, peach, cherry, and hazelnut
Grasses with potato
Ragweed with banana and melons

References: Greer
Laboratories

Please note: This list is for educational use only. Please consult your physician regarding the issue of food cross allergies. Not everyone who develops latex allergy develops cross allergies to foods.

IN THE UNITED STATES DISTRICT COURT
FOR THE EASTERN DISTRICT OF PENNSYLVANIA

IN RE: LATEX GLOVER PRODUCTS: MDL DOCKET NO. 1148

LIABILITY LITIGATION:

: ALL CASES

DAUBERT ORDER- MEMORANDUM

AND NOW, this 10th day of May 2002, defendant manufacturers and distributors of latex gloves having moved *in limine* to exclude the Fed. R. Civ. P. 702 opinion (1) of plaintiffs' witnesses and hearings having been held on February 11-13, March 4-5, and April 22, 2002 the following Daubert rulings are entered: (2)

M. Eric Gershwin, M. D. – Dr. Gershwin, a board certified specialist in allergy, immunology, and internal medicine, is Professor of Medicine and Chief of the Division of Rhenumatology/Allergy and Clinical Immunology at the University of California School of Medicine, Davis, California and is also Chairperson of the Graduate Group in Immunology: No objection was made to his qualification (3)

Opinions 1 through 5(4) – motion denied.

Opinion 5 (each and every exposure to NRL contributes to sensitization and allergy) – motion granted (5) However, the witness is not precluded from testifying to the foundations and reasons given for this opinion.

2. Charles H. Kyper – Mr. Kyper, president of Kyper & Association, a medical device-consulting firm, was employed at the FDA from 1966 to 1994 most recently as Associate Directory for Regulatory Affairs in the Division of Small Manufacturers Assistance and as Assistant Director for

Reclassification and Compliance in the Office of Device Evaluation. The Objections to this witness's qualifications are overruled.(6)

Opinion 1 through 4 (that latex glove manufacturers and distributors were subject to statutory and regulatory obligations sot inform healthcare workers of the risks of glove use, including the giving of timely warnings of the dangers of Type 1 hypersensitivity reactions; that their claims as to hypoallergenicity were misleading: and that they had a duty to report incidents to the FDA showing the potential for serious injury or death arising form glove use) – motion denied. However, unless properly predicated under Fed. R. Civ. P. 703, the witness's hearsay testimony as to issues will be excluded as incompetent.

3. Lawrence J. Broutman, Sc.D. – Dr. Broutman is president of Bodycote Broutman, Inc., a materials testing form, and is Research Professor in the Department of Metallurgical and Materials Engineering at the Illinois Institute of Technology, Chicago, Illinois. The objections to this witness's qualifications are overruled. (7)

Opinions 1 through 3 (8) – motion denied (7)

Edmund V. Ludwig. J.

1.The opinions in question are generic and not case-specific.
2.These general ruling will be supplemented with adjudication as necessitated. The principles of the law and the gatekeeping function of the trial judge are set forth in Daubert v. Merrell Dow Pharm. Inc., 509 U.S. 579, 589, 113 S. Ct. 2786, 2795, 125 L.Ed2d 469 (1993) ("trial judge must ensure that any and all scientific testimony or evidence admitted is not only relevant, but reliable"). A non-exhaustive list of factors is discussed and analyzed.
3.Defendants' three rebuttal witnesses: H. James Wedner, M.D., a specialist in allergy, immunology, and internal medicine, is Professor of Medicine and Director of the Allergy and Immunology Fellowship Training Program at Washington University School of Medicine, St. Louis, Missouri; Steven L. Kagen, M.D., a board certified specialist in allergy, immunology, and internal medicine, is Assistant Clinical Professor in the Division of Allergy and Clinical Immunology at the Medical College of Wisconsin, Professor of Medicine at Department of Community and Family Medicine at Dartmouth Medical School and Director of Cancer Etiology at Norris

Cotton Cancer Center. No objection was made to the qualifications of these witnesses.

4.The options challenged: (1) NRL glove exposure increases the risk of sensitization of allergy; (2) health care workers who wear NRL gloves are at an increased risk for sensitization allergy; (3) powdered NRL gloves increase the risk of sensitization or allergy in comparison with non-powdered gloves; (4) the level of protein or allergen in an NRL glove is associated with the risk of sensitization or allergy; and (5) a dose-response relationship exists between latex glove use and the development of sensitization.

5.This ruling also applies to defendants' joint motion in *limine* to exclude Dr. Gershwin's MDL expert report opinion 8 (Each and every exposure to natural rubber latex gloves manufactured without procedures to reduce water extractable proteins and allergen untis to a low level contributes to sensitization"

6.No witnesses were presented in rebuttal of Mr. Kyper's testimony.

7.Defendants' rebuttal witness was Donald R. Uhlmann, Ph.D., Professor Materials Science and Engineering and of Optical Sciences at the University of Arizona, where he is also Director of the Arizona Materials Laboratory.

8.The challenged opinions: (1) NRL gloves are defective if the manufacturer did not reduce extractable proteins or allergens to the lowest technically and economically feasible level; (2) whether and, if so, when a reasonable manufacturer knew or should have known of the allergic response caused by

Gloves with extractable proteins or allergens and, accordingly, should have changed its manufacturing process; and (3) the extent to which, if any, protein levels in NRL gloves in excess o f specified levels adversely affect barrier protection.

9.Dr. Broutman's testimony is admissible subject to the parties' stipulation that he will not testify to 'medical expert opinion,' including opinions as to 'what levels of protein or allergens in a glove.' (1) 'cause the glove to be capable of causing latex sensitization and or allergy.' (2) cause sensitization or allergy in general; or (3) are safe or unsafe either in a glove or in general. Stipulation 4/9/02 at1.

IN THE UNITED STATES DISTRICT COURT
FOR THE EASTERN INSTRICT OR PENNSYLVANIA
IN RE: LATEX GLOVES PRODUCTS LIABLITY
LITIGATION
MDL DOCKET NO: 1148 ALL CASES

MEMORANDUM

Ludwig. J. August 22, 2001

On the ground of lack of personal jurisdiction, defendant allegiance Corporation moves to be dismissed from all cases excepting those commended in Illinois, where it is headquartered and Delaware, where it is incorporated. Fed. R. Civ. P 12(b)(2). Subject matter jurisdictions diversity. 28 U.S.C. The motion will be denied. These are products liability actions in which plaintiffs, who are medical and hospital professionals and workers, are alleged to have developed toxics reactions from exposure to latex gloves. See Conditional Transfer Order, Fed. 26, 1997. About 500 cases have now been consolidated in this district for coordinated pretrial proceedings, 28 U.S. C. & 1407. (1) At issue here is whether Allegiance Corporation, as a parent company of latex glove manufacturers and distributors, both domestic and foreign, has sufficient contacts with any forum other than Illinois and Delaware to be subject to personal jurisdiction elsewhere.

I BACKGROUND (2)

In 1996, Allegiance Corporation (AC) was incorporated under Delaware law as subsidiary of _____ International Inc., a developer of medical technologies and manufacturer of healthcare product. (2) Joint statement 17

For the purpose of the relevant dates in this case, the following is not is\n dispute. Many managerial functions of AC, AHC, and AHII are performed in a central office located in McGaw Park, Illinois. (6) Id. 37 Acs board of directors meets frequently and acts on financial projects of its subsidiaries, including making loans from AC's lines of credit. Id 38, 78, 85-86. On a number of occasions AC's consist of the same three members who work together regularly, but do not hold in-percent board meetings; instead they transact business in writing. Id 64, 69, 79.

AC has about 50 employees; it subsidiaries employ, altogether, approximately 19, 800. Id 19, 35 AC and AHC share a payroll department, which uses separate bank accounts. Id 47, Healthcare benefits of AC's employees are provided by AHC. ID 45.

Financial statements for AC and to subsidiaries are consolidated, as were its annual shareholder reports when AC was publicly owned Id 81-83

IN THE UNITED STATES DISTRICT COURT
FOR THE EASTERN DISTRICT OF PENNSYLVANIA
IN RE: LATEX GLOVES PRODUCTS LIABILITY
LITIGATION
MDL DOCKET NO. 1148: ALL CASES

MEMORANDUM

Ludwig. J. August 22, 2001

On the ground of lack of personal jurisdiction, defendant Allegiance Corporation moves to be dismissed from all cases excepting those commenced in Illinois, where it is headquartered, and Delaware, where it is incorporated. Fed. R. Civ. P. 12(b)(2). Subject matter jurisdiction is diversity. 28 U.S.C. & 1332. The motion will be denied. These are products liability actions in which plaintiffs, who are medical and hospital professionals and workers, are alleged to have developed toxic reactions from exposure to latex gloves. See Conditional Transfer Order, Fred. 26, 1997. About 500 cases have now been consolidated in this district for coordinated pretrial proceedings, 28. U.S.C & 1407, (1) At issue here is whether Allegiance Corporation, as parent company of latex glove manufacturers and distributors, both domestic and foreign, has sufficient contacts with any forum other than Illinois and Delaware to be subject to personal jurisdiction elsewhere.

I BACKGROUND (2)

In 1996, Allegiance Corporation (AC) was incorporated under Delaware law as a subsidiary of _____ International Inc., a developer of medical technologies and manufacturer of healthcare products. (3) Joint statement 1-2. On September 15, 1996, under an "Agreement and Plan of Reorganization," _____ International transferred t healthcare products assets to AC, including manufacturing and selling of latex gloves. (4) Id 2,6-8. Following the spin-off, AC was a publicly held company until 1999, when it was acquired by Cardinal Health, inc. Id. 12. AC is qualified to do business only in Illinois and Delaware. Id 13.

AC owns 100 percent of the stock of Allegiance Healthcare Corporation (AHC) and Allegiance Healthcare International Inc. (AHII). Id 14, 16, subsidiaries of AHC and AHII manufacture latex gloves and sell them to AHC for marketing and distribution in the United States. (5) Id. 17; Meyers dep. At 31-31, 42. AHC, which owns 50 distribution centers in the United States, does not challenge personal jurisdiction Joint statement 17.

For the purpose of the relevant dates in this case, the following is not in dispute. Many managerial functions of AC, AHC, and AHII are performed in a central office located in McGaw Park, Illinois. (9) Id. 37. AC's board of directors meets frequently and acts on financial projects of its subsidiaries including making loans from AC's lines of credit. Id 38,78, 85-86. On a number of occasions AC's board has bought or sold assets for a subsidiary. Id 77. The boards of directors of AHC and AHII each consist of the same three members who work together regularly, but do not hold in-person board meetings; instead they transact business in writing. Id. 64, 69.79.

AC has about 50 employees; its subsidiaries employ, altogether, approximately
19, 800. Id 19. 35. AC and AHC share a payroll department which uses separate bank accounts. Id 47. Healthcare benefits of AC's employees are provided by AHC. Id. 45.

Financial statements for AC and its subsidiaries are consolidated, as were its annual shareholder reports when AC was publicly owned. Id. 81-83.

II DISCUSSION

Plaintiffs present three theories: (1) the relationship between AC and AHC confers general jurisdiction under alter-ego principles. (8) (2) AC assumed liability for latex gloves claims as part of its spin-off from ____ ___International Inc., citing In re Silicone Gel Breast Implants Products Liability Litigation, in which nationwide jurisdiction was found over ____ ___ International Inc. Based on its merger with American Hospital Supply Corporation, and (3) AC's business activities conducted over the Internet ("www.allegiance.net") establish both general and specific jurisdiction.(9)

Factors three and four –AC and its subsidiaries project a unified marketing image as a single company. Example: on October 1, 1996, a notice in "The Wall Street Journal" pertaining to AC's spin-off from _____ announced in part, as follows

One great company just became two. _____ International is a global leader in the development of medical technologies that save and improve lives around the world. Allegiance Corporation just became America's largest supplier of health-care products and cost-management services for hospitals and other health-care providers. They provide more than 80% of hospital supplies everything from surgical kits and diagnostic equipment to surgeons' gloves and test tubes.

B D A
Business Development Asia

Asian Health Newsletter
Issue 20, August 2000

Focus
The medical glove industry in Malaysia

Malaysia is the world's leading producer of high quality latex gloves, particularly both surgical and examination gloves. They have suffered from an insufficient supply of raw materials, and high cost of labor. The foreign investors had to shift investments and relocate to more favorable countries like Thailand. Thailand is now the second largest rubber glove manufactory, with a 20% share of the market. It is expect to overtake Malaysia in the production of rubber gloves by 2002, as the raw material soppy is sufficient and the labor cost is low. Indonesia is number three with a 10% market share. Over 90% of products produced in Malaysia and Thailand are for export. Malaysia and Thailand together exported 33 billons pairs of gloves.

M & A activity involving foreign parties has been high in both in the rubber glove industry. Allegiance Healthcare, a major US medical equipment provider, has two facilities in Malaysia an on in Thailand that produce rubber gloves. Ansell International, the rubber gives and condoms are of Australia's Pacific Dunlop Ltd, acquired Thai examination glove a condom maker Surtax Group in 1998 and the US-based Johnson & Johnson's global medical glove operation in 1999. In Q1 2000 Kimberly-Clark, the top US maker of personal paper products acquired Safeskin Corp, a San Diego-based disposable latex examination glove maker that has manufacturing facilities in Thailand. Semperit of Austria has a JV manufacturing plant with Sri Trang Agro Industry in Thailand to produce its medical and protective gloves.

Asia Pacific Latex Bhd – established in 1988, the company manufactures powdered and powdered-free gloves under the brand names, Safety & Comfort, Mazpro, Muti Comfort, Polygel, Amerglp and Comfort Star T for overseas market. It is one of the top five latex gloves manufacturers in Malaysia, exporting 88% of its products to the US through US marketing arms, Norwell International Inc. and Asia Pacific Health Care Corporation Inc. It sells the remaining 12 % to Europe via Latech Elastomer Vertriebs in Germany. The company has four manufacturing facilities in Malaysia, with total production capacity of 3 billions gloves per year. It recorded 1999 revenues of Rm 112m (US$30m) and is expected to list on the KLSE in Q4 2000.

Latex Partners Berhad (LPB) – formerly know as Taiping Super Holding BHd, LPB was listed on the KLSE in 1996. It manufactures pre-powdered and powder-free rubber latex glove, for use in medical examination, diagnostic and therapeutic procedures, as well as in dentistry, high-tech manufacturing and food-processing. The annual production capacity of 900 million pre-powder-free gloves of which it can convert 420 millions to powder-free gloves. LPB distributes it own brand of gloves, which are Medtexx, Cleantexx, Techtexx and Dentexx. It recorded 1999 revenues of RM (US 17m).

Top Glove Sdn Bhd established in 1991, Top Glove is the third largest rubber glove manufacturer in Malaysia. It has five factories, which have a total of production capacity of 24 billion gloves per year. The company sells it products in more than 100 counties worldwide.

WRP Asia Pacific And Bhd (WRP) formerly known as Wembley Rubber Products, WRP is one of the three largest manufactures of rubber gloves in the world. The company has an annual production capacity of 4 billion gloves and it running at 80% capacity. WRP reported 1999 revenues of RM350m (US92m) and is planning to list on KLSE in 2002.

YTY Industry Sdn Bhd established in 1989, the company is part of YTY Group that manufactures disposable latex examination gloves Malaysia 3i, an international venture capital firm, led a RM110m (US$29m) management buy-out of YTY Group, giving 3i a substantial minority equity stake YTY Industry operates two facilities in Malaysia with a total production capacity of 1.2 billion gloves. The company sells its products worldwide.

ABOUT BDA

Business Development Asia is a corporate finance advisory firm, which assists US companies to expand their businesses in Asia. BDA specializes in the health industry, helps clients to find local business partners, and has senior advisors in Bangkok, Jakarta, Kuala, Lumpur, Manila, Seoul and Shanghai.

bda@bdallc.com
www.bdallc.com

Marion Ronee Daney

Glossary of Terms
The glossary explains some of the terms related to glove manufacture and allergy issues

Absorbable Dusting Powder (ADP) - A U.S.P. glove donning powder consisting of cornstarch powder mixed weigh approximately 2 percent magnesium oxide to prevent caking. When applied to the surfaces of medical and surgical gloves, it faceplates donning and prevents glove surfaces from sticking together. ADP may be unintentionally deposited into the body during operations or procedures. It is typically absorbed into the body after about three months; however, before it is fully procedures. It is typically absorbed into the body after about three months; however, before it is fully absorbed. ADP may cause the formation of adhesions and granulomas, which can result in serious medical complications.

Accelerator - A chemical that is added to natural rubber latex to help accelerate curing. Thiurams is the most common class of accelerator used in medical glove manufacturing. Other common accelerators include thioureas, mercapto-benzothiazoles, and dithiocarbamates.

Adhesion - An inflammatory band that abnormally joins two tissues or organs by a fibrous growth, especially the opposing surfaces of a wound. Over time, adhesions constrict organs and cause tremendous pain and other complications. Adhesions may form as a post-operative complication of cornstarch powder deposited in body cavities and wounds following surgery.

Allergy - Hypersensitivity caused by exposure to a particular antigen) such as a latex protein or chemical) resulting in a marked increase in relativity to that antigen upon repeated exposure. Sometimes results in harmful immunologic consequences.

Antigen - A foreign substance; an allergen once it has been absorbed into the body and identified by the immune system.

Antibodies - Produced by the body's immunological response to antigens, antibodies are a type of protein found the blood.

Anaphylactic Shock - Systemic response to an allergen resulting in respiratory difficulties and a sudden drop in blood pressure that may lead to cardiovascular collapse. This type of responses may occur in people with Type 1 latex sensitivity.

Atopic - Individuals who are predisposed to allergies in general. Atopic individuals are more likely to develop latex protein allergy than non-atopic individuals.

Chlorination - The process of treating natural rubber with chlorine to improve the donning properties. Chlorination is used in lieu of cornstarch powder in many powder-free gloves.

Contact Dermatitis - A Type IV allergy or irritant reaction characterized by a red rash on the back of the hands and between the fingers. The skin may also develop blisters.

ELISA Assay- Enzyme linked immunosorbent assay, a laboratory test for determining the quantity of soluble proteins represented in latex product extracts.

Antitoxins - Poisons (toxins) remaining after bacteria are broken down during the sterilization of gloves by gamma irradiation. Antitoxins on glove surfaces may lead to skin breakdown and infection, and may cause severe hand dermatitis among healthcare workers.

Granuloma - A nodular inflammatory lesson; usually small or granular, firm, persistent and containing compactly grouped mononuclear blood cells. May be produced by insoluble foreign bodies, such as absorbable dusting powder.

Immunoglobulin E - (IgE) A type of antibody that releases histamines during an allergic reaction. May be triggered by proteins or other allergens.

Inflammation - A process that occurs in blood vessels and adjacent tissues in response to an injury or abnormal physical, chemical or biological stimulation. Signs of inflammation include redness, heat, swelling pain. Inflammation may be caused by latex protein allergy.

Latex- Natural substance produced by the Hevea braillensis (rubber) tree.

Latex Allergy -The body's allergic reaction to one or more of the proteins or added chemical found in natural rubber latex.

LEAP Assay - Latex ELISA for Antigenic Protein, 1 a test to determine the level of latex allergens continued in a product sample. This sensitive test not only measures total latex protein but also measures immunologically reactive protein.

Leaching - Manufacturing process of removing soluble contents of a substance by immersing to water. Latex proteins and chemicals may be removed form latex products during the leaching and rinsing stages of manufacturing.

Lowery Assay - A method of testing for the level of total latex protein contained in a product sample.

Lypcopodium - The spores of the club moss. When processed, it becomes a yellow, tasteless and colorless powder. Lycopodium was once used as a dusting powder on medical gloves, but abandoned after it was proven to remind in the body and cause inflammatory responses and other serious medical complications.

Pyrogen - Bacteria, molds, viruses and years that cause fever. Pyrogens can remains on gloves following sterilization by gamma irradiation.

Universal Precautions - Glove guidelines for healthcare workers mandated by the U.S. Centers for Disease Control and Prevention in 1987 to help prevent the transmission of HIV.

RAST Inhibition Test - Radioallergosorbent laboratory test which indicates the amount of allergens present in a glove extract.

Sensitivity - A term used in assessing the value of a diagnostic test, procedure or clinical observation. It is the proportion of people who truly have a specific disease and are so identified by the test.

Sensitivity - A condition of being made susceptible to a specific substance such as protein or pollen by repeated exposure over a period of time. Sensitization is the precursors to allergy.

Talc - Hydrous magnesium silicate, used as dusting powder. Abandoned as a substance of donning gloves because it was proven to cause inflammatory responses and other severe medical complication when deposited in the body during surgery.

Vulcanization - The process of treating raw rubber or its compounds by subjecting it to heat in the presence of sulfur to increase its strength and elasticity.

RESOURCE PAGE

Medicine's Deadly Dust, A Surgeon's Wake-up Call to Society

Richard F. Edlich, M. D., Ph.D. with Juliea A. Woods and Mary Jude Cox

Published by Vandamere Press, Arthur Brown (Publisher),

P.O. Box 5243, Arlington, VA 22205, Copyright 1997

vandamere@netzero.com

References pages used- 65,66,67,73,74,75,76,77,78,79.83,88,109,110,116,117,121,

122,123,124,125, 130,131

Latex Allergy In Neurosurgical Practice
Division of Neurosurgery
Children's Hospital of Eastern Ontario-Canada
By Mazagri R: Ventureyra EC
Childs Nerv Syst (CNV0, 1999 AUG 15 (8) : 404-2
Record: 99376788
JOURNAL ARTICLE: REVIEW: REVIEW, TUTORIAL
http://firstsearch.oclc.org//:next

Patient Care, Feb 15, 1996 v30 n3 p32, Latex allergy: potentially dialing. *Nancy Walsh D'Epiro, COPYRIGHT Medical Economics Publishing 1996*

June 1997, DHHS (NIOSH) Publication No. 97-135, ALERT- Preventing Allergic Reactions to Natural Rubber Latex in the Workplace, p. 5

Latex Allergy: potentially disabling. Nancy Walsh D'Patient Care, Feb 15, 1996 v30n3p32 (3) COPYRIGHT Medical Economics Publishing 1996, L Epiro.

June 1997, DHHS (NIOSH) Publication No. 97-135, ALERT- Preventing Allergic Reactions to Natural Rubber Latex in the Workplace, p. 5

RAST update
IMVS Newsletter Number 46 Winter 2002

By David Gillis
www.imvs.so.gov.au

Germans Allergists Develop Breakthrough Test
The Week in Germany: Business and Technology
September 24, 2004
http://www.germanyinfo.org/relaunch/info/publications//
week/2004/04094/economy2.html

LEAP Testing Service
Email: LTS@guthrie.org

Diagnosis
SKINmed 2(6): 359-366, 2003 © 2003 Le Jacq Communications, Inc.

Latex Allergy test Discern Which Patients Need Avoidance Management:
Presented at AAAAI
Microarray-based Improvement of Diagnosis for Latex Allergy. Abstract 442
By Paula Moyer
http://www.docguide.com/news/content.nsf/news/
8525697700573E1885256FCD0063414…

© 1997, London International Group plc, all rights reserved, site developed by Acumen Solutions. http;//www.regentmedical.com/uk_rgent/summslav.htm
Patient Care, Feb 15, 1996 v30n3p32(3) COPYRIGHT Medical Economics Publishing 1996 "Latex is the allergen of the '90s.(p.3 in the article

JUNE 1997, DHHS (NIOSH) Publication No. 97-135- ALERT- PREVENTING ALLERGIC REATIONS TO NATURAL RUBBER LATEX IN THE WORKPLACE, p. 5

Reprinted from Medical Sciences Bulletin, published by Pharmaceutical Information Associated, Ltd.(MSB:- Medical Sciences Bulletin Contents) (PIA: - Pharmaceutical Information Associates Homepage) (PIN: - PharmInfoNet Homepage)

Marion Ronee Daney

The Wall Street Journal, Oct 1, 1997n196pB11(W)pB17(E)col4(4col in)JUNE 1997, DHHS (NIOSH) Publication No. 97-135- ALERT-PREVENTING ALLERGIC REATIONS TO NATURAL RUBBER LATEX IN THE WORKPLACE, p. 5

Facts About latex Allergies
Latex Allergy Fact Sheet
Latex Allergy is an acquired Allergy
© 2000 Andover Coated Products
http://www.andovercoated.com/nolatex/fact_sheet.html

Latex Hazards
Contact Information: Phone: (708) 760-6558 Email: The Magical Balloon-dude Dale. http://www.ecn.bgu.edu/users/gdobro/Hazars. html

Reprinted from Medical Sciences Bulletin, published by Pharmaceutical Information Associated, Ltd.(MSB:- Medical Sciences Bulletin Contents) (PIA: - Pharmaceutical Information Associates Homepage) (PIN: - PharmInfoNet Homepage)

© 1993-1999 Microsoft Corporation. All rights reserved, "Softball," pg. 1

(U.S. Food and Drug Administration) [FDA Home Page]

Mouth   piece   by   Douglas   Hoffman,   MD **http;//www.allhealth.com/conditions/allergies/qa/0,4801,41_ 176068,00html**

Gum chewing

Microsoft ® Encarta ® Encyclopedia 2000 © 1993-1999 Microsoft Corporation.

Something Was Not Right About David!
Children Reactions
The Canadian and Americans Latex Associations1`1`
By Karen

http://www.allergicchild.com/latex_allergies.htm

Children On Home Mechanical Ventilation At Risk For Latex Allergy
A Doctor's Guide Review of: "Latex Allergy in Children on Home Mechanical
Ventilation
By David Loshak 10-23-2000
http;//www.doc.guide.com/news

Can Pacifiers and Diapers Trigger Allergies in Infants?
NEW YORK (Rueters Health) September 30, 1999
SOURCE ALLERGY 1999;541007
Copyright 1999 Reuters Limited
http://www.intelihealth.com
Pacifiers Do Have A Positive Side
The Use Of Pacifiers and SIDS
Allergy 1999; 54:1007 Reuter Limited Copyright 1999

May 2000 © 2000 by Medscape Inc. All rights reserved. Anne Scheck is a
freelance medical writer.

Safe, Latex-Free Condoms: Ending an Unpleasant Allergy Reaction?
By Anne Scheck, Medical Writer

http;//healthwatch.medscape.com/medscape/p/G_Library/article.
asp?RecID=215375&Cont...

New York Daily News Sunday June 13, 1999 by Susan Ferraro
Physicians Against Latex Sensitization[PALS]
http;//www.barbarazuckerpinchoff.com/pals/press.htm
http://www.findarticles.com/cf_0/m0UMR/12_20/58239066/pl/article.
jhtml

http://www.mambaby.com/englisch/mam_english_s16c.html

ALLERGY HAZARD
Growing number of health care workers developing dangerous reaction to
latex
The Patriot Ledger Tues, April 1, 1997
By Liz Kowalczyk

Marion Ronee Daney

http://latexallergylinks.tripod.com/ledger.html

Latex Allergy News Introductory Issue 1997,www.latexallergyhelp.com
176 Roosevelt Avenue, Torrington, CT 06790

How Can A Child Life be Disrupted?
A Child's Perspective By Douglas, Pennsylvania
http://www.latexallergyhelp.com/child.htm

The American Medical Association News, October 13, 1997, Vol. 40, Number 38,
By Margaret Veach - AMNEWS CORRESPONDENT

Local women lives in fear

Dailey News by Terrence Synnott

Copyright © 1996-2001 Elastics Inc. Revised on Sun March 11, 2001

http://www.latex-allergy.org/Hatl.html -.

http://www.harbourhealth.com/scripts/om.dll/serve?action=searchDB&searchDBfor=art&a...

BEACON- A Publication Of The Alumni Association Of New Jersey Dental School
beacon.ac-lates1 - http;//www.umdnuj.edu/njdsaweb/beac.v1.latex.html

Latex Allergy Awareness Week
http://www.latex-allergy.org/RI.html
Copyright © 1996-2001 ELASTIC Inc.
Revised on Sun Mar 11 2001

Pat Lawson is the ELASTIC state representative for Iowa

http://www.latex-allergy.org/iowa.html

© 2000 The Morning Call Inc.
http;//gelmans.com/Focus/21/5/page5.html
Focus on the Law, June 1999 Volume 21,#5

http://www.bizjournals.com/buffalo/stories/2000/01/31/daily17.html

This article is © The Morning Call Newspaper Company, Tuesday, November 16, 1999
Pg. A01 Edition: FIFTH Section: NATIONAL - by Diane Marczely Gimpel, The Morning Call

Copyright © 1997 by The Finley Hospital. All rights reserved
http://www.finleyhospital.org/housecalls/Mar00/Story5.htm

http://qctimes, com/rednews/1999/12/08/build/local/STOPY4.html
By Ross Bielama, QUAD-CITY TIMES- December 8, 1999

http://www.regentmedical.com/uk-rgent/gloossary.htm

Anaphylaxis Reports
Departments of Anesthesiology, Surgery, Division of Pediatric Surgery and Nursing
University of Virginia Health Sciences Center
P.O. Box 10010, Charlottesville, VA 22908 http://gasnet.med.yale.edu//esia/1997/december/
Educational Synopses in Anesthesiology and Criticall Care Medicine Vol.4 No 12

http://gasnet.med.yale.edu//esia/1997/december/
Educational Synopses in Anesthesiology and Criticall Care Medicine Vol.4 No 12

Please send correspondence to Burhard F. Spiekermann, MD
E-mail: BTS4C@Virginia.edu
Tel: 804-924-2203 fax: 804-982-0019

Natural Rubber Latex Allergy: A Potentially Disabling Epidemic
By Rochelle D. Spiker, MSW, LCSW-C
Executive Director of the Potomac Latex Allergy Association
Tel. 341-567-1559 Fax: 314-567-5552
paraquad@paraquad.org

Attention: Health, Industrial and forward planning editors
100,000 NHS staff allergic to gloves designed to protect
July 30, 2001

Marion Ronee Daney

All TUC press releases can be found at www.tuc.org.uk
Media enquiries: Stephanie Power: spower@tuc.org.uk

Greendale Firefighter claims Disability, blaming Latex
Milwaukee-Journal Sentinel Staff
By Kenneth R. Lamke`
December 16, 1997
© Copyright 1999, Milwaukee Journal Sentinel

http://wwwjsonline.com/archive/dec97/news/metro/
971216greendalefirefighterc.stm

R | D Group study on 27 cases with latex allergy
Ritsuko Hayakawa*,
Research Group for New Material of Rubber Products
*Department of Environmental Dermatology, Nagoya University School of
Medicine,
http://allergy.nch.go.jp/latex/V2-1/24.htm

Warning on Hospital Gloves:
Koop Criticized for Role in Warning on Hospital Gloves
By Holcomb B. Noble, The New York Times National
Friday, October 29, 1999

Journal of Respiratory Diseases, April 2002 v23 i4 p250 (7)
Is occupational latex allergy causing your patient's asthma?
Hives and "hay fever" symptoms are common warning signs.
B. Lauren Charous; Margaret A. Charous. COPYRIGHT 2002 Cliggott
Publishing Co (Health Reference Center-Academic-Article 14 of 192)

The Ultimate EMS Resource
http://www.merginet.com/index.efm?pg=wellness&fn=latexallergy
webmaster@merginet.com

SOURCE Food Allergy & Anaphylaxis Network Web Site: http://www.
foodallergy.org.
http://foodallergy.org/advocacy.html#emt
Issues of news releases and not PR Newswire are solely responsible for the
accuracy for the contents. Terms and conditions, including on redistribution,
apply

The Food Allergy & Anaphylaxis Network, 11781 Lee Jackson Hwy. Suite 160,
Fairfax, VA 22033, (1-800-929-4040) www.foodallergy.org
©Copyright 2005

http:www.smileon.com/news/news_view.php?news_id=2020
©Smile-on Ltd 2005
editor@amile-on.com.

Latex nipple. (On formula bottles could caused infant allergy (Brief Article)
Pediatrics for Parents, April 2002 v20i4p2(1)
Full Text: COPYRIGHT 2002 Pediatrics for Parents. Inc.
Annals of Emergency Medicine 4/02.
This database brought to you by, Heath Reference Center Academic
http://web7.infotrac.galegroup.com/itw/informark/149/832/42672506w7/pul=rcl_HRCA-

Lip, Swollen (Allergic Reaction). B.D. Schmitt
Clinical Reference System, Annual 2001 p1202
Full Text: COPYRIGHT 2001 McKesson Health Solutions LLC

Oregon soon to ban latex glove use: foodservice workers will not be allowed to use latex rubber gloves beginning in March 2003. (Small is Beautiful)
Scott Human. Restaurants & Institutions, Oct 15, 2002 v112 i23 p.78 (1)
Full Text: COPYRIGHT 2002, Reed Business information.
Copyright© 2003 by Gale Group. All rights reserved. Gale Group is a Thomson-Corporation Company.

Official allergen list by WHO-OUIS
Allergen nomenclature Allergen sequence database (BISF)
Allergen sequence database (BISF)
Monthly journal indexing on allergens and related articles (ISFA)
NIHS/DMD/yagam@nihs.go.jp
htttp://dmd.nihs.go.ap/latex/allergen-e.html

Marion Ronee Daney

Update on the Law...
Latex Allergy Litigation
By Jon. L. Gelman {1}
Volume 21, Issue 7 November 1999
http://www.gelmans.com/Articles/latexsurvey99/latexsurvey11991.htm

LATEX ALLERGY NEWS
Volume VI issue 5
June1999
ISSN (SSN#1084-1121)

Elastic - Education for Latex Allergy / Support Team & Information Coalition
Lethal Latex
http://www.latex-allergy.org/texas/html
By Carolyn Porot Staff Writer, Star Telegram, Wed. Dec. 18, 1996, reproduced here with permission.
http://www.latex-allergy/texas.html
Copyright © 1996-2001 ELASTIC Inc.
Revised on Sun Mar 11, 2001

TATTOO SANTA BARBARA. (805) 968-7552
Pat Fish
318 State Street, Santa Barbara, CA 93101-2361 USA
http://www.luckyfish.net/glovealert.html

Rotavirus infection in children with acute diarrhea as detected by latex agglutination, ``ELISA and polyacrylamide gel electrophoresis.
Authors: Altindis M: Yavrou SL Simsek A; Ozkul A: Ceri A: Koc H
Affiliation: Kocatepe University School of medicine, Department of Microbiology and Clinic Microbiology, Afyon, Turkey
ISSN: 0019-6061;NLM Unique Journal Identifier: 2985062R
MEDLINE
maltindis@hotmail.com

FirstSearch® Copyright © 1992-2004 OCLC as to electronic and platform
All Right Reserved http://FirstSearch.oclc.org

Increased prevalence of latex-sensitization among children with chronic renal failure.
Authors: Dehlink E; Prandstetter C; Eiweggrt T; Urbanek R; Szepfalusi Z,

Affiliation: Department of Pediatrics, Division of General Pediatrics, Medical University of Vienna, Vienna, Austria
FirstSeach® copyright © 1992-2004 OCLC as to electronic presentation and platform
FirstSearch@oclo.org Location: http://FirstSearch.oclc.org

C. A. Reject Manufacturing-Defect Finding in First Latex Glove Trial
Fourth District Panel Says It Was Reasonable for Maker to Weigh One Safety Consideration Against Another
Metropolitan News-Enterprise: By Kenneth Ofgang, Staff Writer/Appellate Courts: Friday 21, 2002
Copyright 2002, Metropolitan News Company
http://www.metnews.com/articles/glov062101.htm

In vivo and vitro in diagnosis of latex allergy at Groote Schuur Hospital
Authors: Marais GI; Fletcher JM; Potter PC
Department of Immunology, Groove Schuur Hospital, Cape Town
Source S Afr Med J (South African medical journal. Suld-Afrikaanse tydskrif vir geneeskunde.)
1997 Aug; 87(8): 1004-8
Additional Info: SOUTH AFRICA
STANDARD NO: ISSN: 0038-2469; NLM Unique Journal Identifier: 0404520

CONDOM INFORMATION
HOW LATEX CONDOMS ARE MADE & TESTED
www.durex.com
http://www.justrubbers.com/info/latex_condom.html

ATTORNEY GENERAL WANT TO BAN LATEX GLOVES IN RHODE ISLAND FOOD INDUSTRY

(The Boston Globe web sit is at http://wwwboston. com/globe/)
PBN COM
Providence Business News
Rhode Island's Premier Business News and Resource Website
http://www.pbn.com/contentmgr/showdetails.php???id=5919

Public Affairs Division

Marion Ronee Daney

National Paint & Coating Association
1500 Rhode Island Ave, N.W.
Washington, D.C. 20005
Phone 202/462-6272
Fax 202/462-0347
Email: npca@paint.org
        NPCA contact: Lisa Warren
        Public Affairs Division

<u>Are Latex and Food allergies Related?</u>
References: Greer Laboratory

IN THE UNITED STATES DISTRICT COURT
FOR THE EASTERN DISTRICT OF PENNSYLVANIA
http://www.paed.uscourts.gov/documents/opinions/01D0689P.
HTM

Poetry

Marion Ronee Daney

<u>The Is My Poetry</u>
<u>Depression Is The Monster That Lives Within Me</u>

Depression is the monster that lives within me
Sometimes I cry so hard that my eyes are swollen
And it seems as though my tears won't stop flowing down my cheeks
In my despair is so convicting that I feel lost and alone
This Monster that I call Depression he takes me by the hand
He takes me to a place where I fall, fall and continue to fall until darkness
surrounds me
I don't even know why he follow me
I don't know how he fines me
But he is there waiting lurking and always ready to devourer me
I don't know how I arrived at this place
Where emptiness just smile at me
Depression has it own mine and spirit
He puts me in a hole where all of the tunnel walls led me to more dark tunnel walls
If I try to climb out there is no ladder or rope to escape
I even try to fight him with my boxing gloves on
But at times his manipulative voice over powers me
So I lose again time after time
I am on my knees praying that this Monster which he calls himself Depression
Leave me alone!
Taunting me in my dreams where I thought that I was safe from being victimize
No! Never! He tells me with a smirk on his face and then he just laughs
He believes that his Wisdom is Great and that he will always have me feeling
pessimistic
I sit alone with silence
Until I hear my heart shatter like a crystal glass
Faith! Faith! I am calling your name
Can you hear me?
Smile at me and show me your Wisdom
Allow me to touch your spirit and embrace intelligence
Look for Love for me
Tell her that I need her light
So my scattered heart can be mended
Then the healing can begin
The Monster Depression will have no place for his Wisdom within me
My heart would then be free like a flower blooming in the Spring time
Awaking from a deep Sleep
Full of Beauty and Love

By Marion Ronee Daney © March 4, 2003

Can the Angels Hear My Soul Crying?

Can the Angels hear my Soul crying?
When I speak words
Will the words vanish into the darkness and not go towards the light
Will all the pain that I have suffered go unnoticed
So many times my despair completely disconnected me from my exists
The tomorrows in my life were just in my dreams
No hopes no promises and the sun seemed like it did not shine
Even the birds expresses whispering in and all around was voids in my heart
Waking up in the morning taking a deep breath and trying to continue the
nightmare
That never seems to end
Walking in the shadow of death was easy for me It was my daily walk
Pretending that my tears was not real
Can the Angels hear my soul crying
It seems as though my heart is cold filled with darkness
I try listening for my heart beating
There is only silence
Love suppose to fine me and save me
Save me and guild me out of the darkness
My soul is trapped in a dark room behind a door
As I open it to find my soul
My soul is just a pile of ash
As I fall to my knees and pray that my soul come back to me
Please embrace me again
Please fine your way back to me
So I won't be hypnotized anymore to stay in the darkness
So I can be free to feel my heart beating again
So I can love
The tears that I cry won't be filled with torment in every drop
For once and forever walk in the love
With every footstep
Allow love to complete who I am
To guide me to my Destiny

Marion Ronee Daney © Feb. 26, 2003

Marion Ronee Daney

My Awaking From A Deep Sleep

My awaking from a deep sleep
In the Fairytale Sleeping Beauty
As the fruit poisoned her
From just one bites she took
Then she fell into a deep sleep
Only to be awakened by a kiss from a True Prince
This Prince had to be full of Love
As the words in the world trampled over me
I too feel into a deep sleep
I had eaten of the World
In which their fruits were poisoning me
I was not mindful at all
I was slipping, slipping, and slipping away
I could not see
Everything was hazy to me
Numbness was all I became
The Sun showed her presence
But I could not envision her gracefulness
The Universe called my name
I did not hearken to her music
They bewitched me in another Universe
Where time seems like it did not exist
Where convictions was not alive
Until It became transparent to me
That I was in bondage
Before a Butter Fly is awaken after the Winter completes her enchanting smile
She is growing from a caterpillar into a mature Butter Fly
She had to take a long journey
From an egg to crawling around eating leaf after leaf
Until it was time to create her jade colored Cocoon
So she had to make it just right so she could survive the Winter's smile
When the Spring approaches Dancing
She the ButterFly knows the sound of the Spring's music playing
She is ready with vibrate sparkling golden colors on her wings with black tear
drops
To show the World that awakening from deep sleep
Can Truly make you Beautiful
If you follow your heart

As I awakened from my deep sleep
I realize that I must be meek

I must open my Heart completely to the Universe
Listen to her Music which is her Wisdom
She will divulge all her Secrets
That will lead me to be Victorious

Marion R, Daney © carch 21, 2003

My White Angel

She was very alluring to me
When she came into my life
My imagination did not know what would be bestowal my journey
She enticed me so compasssionaltely
I felt her the White Angel took me to heaven
My whole boy surrendered and absorbed into
Her consciousness and her being
I was then lost without her touch of joy that I felt every time
She became one with my substance
My realities seem no more
As long as I knew her tenderness was with me
All the money that I worked for was for her
Although I knew that I could lose everything
So damn what!
My friends no more
My family no more
My job hanging by a tread
A disaster waiting to happen
But my nose is very lonely
I just have to have my White Angel to rescue me
My only hope of being complete again
Just another snort
I say! I say! I say!
Even when my head is spinning
Oh please stop!
Maybe I am Alice in Wonderland
Hey! Maybe I am A Cinderella
And I am waiting for Prince Charming's lush's kiss
But my nose will not stop bleeding
And my heart will not stop beating so rapidly
Nobody can touch me like this!
My White Angel! My White Angel I need her seducing smile
She drives me wild and I love every exciting moment that she brings
My White Angel promised me her white feathery wings

So I would fly free forever and ever
My White Angel promised me that she would never forsake me
Now, I am crying and crying

I know that my White Angel only gave me empty promises
Now my soul I cannot fell it anymore
Now my heart I cannot hear the beat
To look at myself it is hard
What have I done?
I thought my White Angel was going to keep me from harm
But all along she captivated me with her wisdom
She deceived me
She devourered me
She took all of me
Now there is none of me left

Written By Marion Ronee Daney © Copywriter 1/97

Marion Ronee Daney

Me And My Shadow's Journey

Me And My Shadow staggering down the street
Since I am the Shadow, my Master enslaves me
Whatever he wishes to do I must follow in his footsteps
Since he calls whiskey his companion and indulges delightfully smiling
As he begins to laugh loudly after taking another big gulp
He looks at me and says, "What is you looking at Shadow?"
Ha! Ha! Ha!, Want some?
Then he asked me, "How do I get home?" "Where am I?"
Hey! I am just your Shadow, "What can I do?"
Now, I know that you are hallucinating and intoxication has set in
Your mind at this time is incoherent and they have totally imbalanced
your visual abilities
But hey you enjoy Sweet Names like Drunk, Boozer, Lush, Alcoholic
Driving is out of the question you are delusional
Your brain is at a shut down
You may not realize that your brain cells are vanishing daily because of
the torture that you Chosen For you
Still, all you say is "Just another drink!" "Just another drink I need to
function!"
Your poor heart is malfunctioning, and your liver is scarred
Me And My Shadows use to have fun without that liquor
So you think that you have many problems and escaping in a bottle is the
answer
Facing reality is not a road that is always easy
But having faith in your self and keeping your dreams alive is a good
place to start
So therefore, you can achieve your true destiny
Drinking can tear down your body tissues and then you decide to binge
it could just kill you
Your life is not the only one affected by your decisions
Drunk Driving ☺ Under the influence of Alcohol for so-called fun
daring circumstances
It can have fatally consequences along the way
Don't allow alcohol to imprison your mind, heart and spirit
Being dependent on alcohol can lead up to Alcoholic Psychosis and
Wernicke's Encephalopathy
It is severe Mental Disorders like Pathologic Intoxication, Delirium Tremens, Acute
Hallucinosis, and Korasakoff's Psychosis brain damage characterizes this

Footsteps are yours to create for your journey of tomorrows
Don't walk in the shadows
Walk in the light ✡

Written by Marion R, Daney ©1-13-99

Marion Ronee Daney

<u>*My Tears will fall Silent*</u>

My tears will fall silent
Only if my voice can not be heard
The tears will fall on my face like a stream
Where will they go?
Will someone catch them before they fall?
Will someone listen before they have a chance to disappear?
Darkness will surround the tears because the are empty and lost
A tear has many stories to tell
Are you willing to listen?
Will you stay and be patient with her
To her story of Betray and Deceit
Her roads that she travel have no path to follow
She just wanders here and there
Consumed in her Despair
Faith will arrive one day and her tears will feel joy
Then she can be content
Love will then guild her
She will no longer be alone and the sun will embrace her.

Marion R, Daney © 1/27/2005

I Am Beautiful Always

I Am Beautiful Always
As I see there is only darkness surrounding me
Suddenly, the sun unveils her presence once again
Graceful when she spreads her love in the universe
With her brilliant light
Miraculously awakens all
Giving us another day of beauty
Just take a deep breathe and smell the sweetness of the pine trees
Indulge yourself into the beauty of the fragrance
When Springtime, arrives just stop for a moment
Visualize that we are all beautiful flowers
That we in our lives have to bloom with perfection
As we spread our arms and grow
They spread their pedals with beauty like the rainbow
There one purpose in their lives is to be truly beautiful
Also to show us we are the same
As the birds from heaven take a flight making the heavens a play ground
It is just breathtaking how they caress the winds
They take charge of their destiny and they know how enjoy in
their spirit
Being totally free
Just fly, fly with loveliness as the wind is beating with the rhythm of their hearts
Beautiful singing their sweet melodies in harmony with each other
As we can truly be a free spirit
Letting love guild us to our destinies
We can fly too
Just listen
Listen, closely to the rain falling and falling
She is whispering love
Can't you hear her?
Now, it is time for nature to be silent
To close her eyes and rest
Until dawn calls her name Beauty
Then she will awaken once more

Marion Daney ©

Marion Ronee Daney

A Touch Of Innocence

A Touch Of Innocence
Sweet as a flower
Beautiful when the flower blooms
The fragrance is like unto pure honey
Wonderful melodies from the small sparrow
Singing his song
Whom has the right to violate the innocence?
Not allowing someone to blossom like the flowers do
The sun will be in her place
But some innocence will be blinded from her light
Where are the roads that the innocence travels?
If the innocence would be robbed of their paths
So then, they would be lost and sometimes forever
Where does hopes exist?
When the innocence only given fear and told lies
Then they won't be able to have faith
Tomorrows suppose to be filled up with promises and dreams
How could it be when they end up with broken promises?
Nightmares that is their daily life
They have to hide it from the world
Pretend that it never happened
When does the innocence be protected from harm?
So that they would be able to be free to laugh and play
The innocence is our tomorrow
If we don't love them
Stand with them
Guide them with all our might
We would then be violating our innocence

Marion Ronee Daney   © 2/97

My True Hero

My true hero
He follows me every where I go
He holds my hand to fill in the void
He walks with me
So I won't walk alone
He keeps me warm at times that I need to be warm
When I need comfort he is there
I make many sacrifices to be with him
As I gaze into his crystalline eyes
I can see my future
He touches my soul
He opens my mind
With a smoothing calming excitement
My stress I don't feel any more
Relieving anxiety
As I slip into a stupor state
My mental numbness arises
Within me
Then I just laugh and laugh
Until what I don't even know
Hey I can't even find a vein
It is some of what painful
That dam hematoma
Just why me?
I need to gaze into his crystalline eyes
I can't deal with those shaking spells
Those hot and cold sweats again
Goose bumps all over my body
Just if I can get him into my veins and feel his sensation
Giving my body a rush
So I can feel his vibrate spirit touching me
I just can't eat I can't sleep
I just hear him calling my sweet name
So now my addictive spit is haunted day and night
By his voice
It is like a nightmare, I am totally trapped
As long as I am submissive to him
He will control my thoughts and who I am
It didn't use to be like this

Marion Ronee Daney

I had control
But now I have nothing
Nothing at all
As it is said look into my crystal ball can it
Really is a mirror to my soul to be

Marion Ronee Daney © *1/97*

SARAH LOVE

SARAH LOVE HAS TOUCHED OUR LIVES
WITH SO MUCH LAUGHTER
AND HER TENDER KISSES
I WILL FEEL NO MORE UPON MY CHEEK
AS SHE WOULD THEN HUG ME SO TIGHT
I COULD HEAR HER HEART BEATING
AGAINST MY CHEST
AND THEN SHE WOULD THEN
WHISPER MY NAME
WHERE ARE THE SWEET DAYS OF
SARAH GONE
WHERE ARE THE STARS
THEY DON'T SPARKLE THE SAME ANY MORE
EVEN THOUGH THE BIRDS CONTINUE TO SING
BUT THE MELODY IS NOT THE SAME
NOW, AS MY TEARS FALL
IT SEEMS LIKE FOREVER
FOR MY SWEET SARAH
TOMORROW IS NO MORE
SOMETIMES I WISH LIFE WAS LIKE
A FAIRYTALE
AS PRINCE CHARMING KISSES SNOW WHITE
ON HER ROSE COLOR LIPS
SHE AWAKENS WITH A DAZZLING SMILE
SARAH CAN ONLY WAKE UP
IN MY DREAMS OF TOMORROW
AND SMILE AT ME

Marion R. Daney © 10-12-96

Marion Ronee Daney

I've Been Dreaming
Dreaming Of You

When I go to sleep at night
I think of only you
I just can't wait
To hold you near
To embrace your tenderness
I've been dreaming
 Dreaming of you
I see that sparkling smile
Your little finger tips and toes
Most of all your soft
Baby doll eyes
I've been dreaming
Dreaming of you
I close my eyes
And I am hugging you
I am rocking you to sleep
I am tucking you in your crib
I am kissing you good night
My Precious
I've Been Dreaming
Dreaming of you
Now, my imagination
Will unfold and be
A beautiful life
That grew inside of me
 A beating heart
A Throbbing Soul existing
I pray that the Spirits
Will protect you
Guide you out of Darkness
Most of all Show you Love
Beyond my Dreams
Of Tomorrow

Marion Ronee Daney
 (c) 1996

MY TRUE HERO

MY TRUE HERO
HE FOLLOWS ME EVERY WHERE I GO
HE HOLDS MY HAND TO FILL IN THE VOID
HE WALKS WITH ME
SO I WON'T WALK ALONE
HE KEEPS ME WARM AT TIMES THAT I NEED TO BE WARM
WHEN I NEED COMFORT HE IS THERE
I MAKE MANY SACRIFICES TO BE WITH HIM
AS I GAZE INTO HIS CRYSTALLINE EYES
I CAN SEE MY FUTURE
AND HE TOUCHES MY SOUL
AND OPENS MY MIND
WITH A SMOOTHING CALMING EXCITEMENT
MY STRESS I DON'T FEEL ANY MORE
RELIEVING ANXIETY
AS I SLIP INTO A STUPOR STATE
MY MENTAL NUMBNESS ARISES
WITHIN ME
THEN I JUST LAUGH AND LAUGH
UNTIL WHAT I DON'T EVEN KNOW
HEY I CAN'T EVEN FIND A VEIN
AND IT IS SOME OF WHAT PAINFUL
THAT DAM HEMATOMA
JUST WHY ME?
I NEED TO GAZE INTO HIS CRYSTALLINE EYES
I CAN'T DEAL WITH THOSE SHAKING SPELLS
THOSE HOT AND COLD SWEATS AGAIN
GOOSE BUMPS ALL OVER MY BODY
JUST IF I CAN GET HIM INTO MY VEINS AND FEEL HIS SENSATION
GIVING MY BODY A RUSH
SO I CAN FEEL HIS VIBRATE SPIRIT TOUCHING ME
I JUST CAN'T EAT I CAN'T SLEEP
I JUST HEAR HIM CALLING MY SWEET NAME
SO NOW MY ADDICTIVE SPIRIT IS HAUNTED DAY AND NIGHT
BY HIS VOICE
IT IS LIKE A NIGHTMARE I AM TOTALLY TRAPPED
AS LONG AS I AM SUBMISSIVE TO HIM
HE WILL CONTROL MY THOUGHTS AND WHO I AM

Marion Ronee Daney

IT DIDN'T USE TO BE LIKE THIS
I HAD CONTROL
BUT NOW I HAVE NOTHING
NOTHING AT ALL
AS IT IS SAID LOOK INTO MY CRYSTAL BALL CAN IT
REALLY BE A MIRROR TO MY SOUL TO BE

MARION RONEE DANEY © 1/97

Say I Am The Driver

Say I am the driver
I am the master of my car
When I put the key in the ignition
I then turn the switch on
And roar my engine up
I talk to my car
I tell her that we are on another journey
I want to return home safe
I try to be conscious of all of my surrounding
At all times
So therefore I do not intake alcohol or any illegal drugs
I let nothing distract my concentration
I respect the road that she is
And I want her to protect me from harm
Sometimes Mother-Nature whispers her tunes like Blizzards, Blinding Sunlight,
Thunder & Lighting Storms, and Harsh Rainy Days
Also don't forget the foggy days and deepest darkest night that creep upon us
Which make the roads very slippery and hard to locate her the road
But I stay in harmony with her
So I would be safe from harm
I realize I am not vincible
I am at her mercy
When I go on her territory
My life is in her hands in a matter of speaking
We as drivers need to stop taking life for granted
Life is very very precious
we only have one chance to do it right
Life could be changed completely and taken away with just a twinkle of an eye
No matter how big you think you are
The harder you can fall
So please stop and think
Your are not on the road by yourself
We must share the road and be courteous
Watch out for children playing, bike riders, pedestrians, and motor cycles, moped,
Going the speed limit is the law it just might save your life
We must respect her
In return she will respect you

Marion Ronee Daney

Protect you from harm
And return you home safely

Marion Ronee Daney © 2-14-97

CONCLUSION

I hope that who ever read this book they did get some understand about latex allergy. I am grateful that I took the time to do this. I was so caught up doing the book I do not remember typing all the words and even doing all the research. It seemed funny it was words that was presented to me. Now all the words came together out of spirit and they made since. Since Latex Allergy was diagnosed, the Food Drug Administration stepped up to the plate and demanded changes. Which the companies were required changes must be. Therefore, now there are latex gloves, which have less cornstarch and some glove are powered-free to prevent sensitizing. There are products now that are latex-free. There are companies that offer different types of gloves that are safe for employers. Some the hospital now use non-powdered latex gloves. Some doctor offices are latex-safe environment for the patients and the working staff. My concerns were about the innocent children that had surgery in the hospitals, there were changes for them. Anaphylactic Shock is no joke; it can be a severe reaction to a bee sting or food. Therefore, if you have any questions or concerns about your medications, food allergies, insect bite, or latex allergies please contact your doctor. If you are allergic to latex, please inform your Doctor or Dentist before any type of procedure and surgery. Remember they do not know if you were tested or had reactions if you do not tell them. Make sure the doctor office put it on your chart and please wear an alert bracelet or necklace of some kind. Just in case if, you have to be admitted to the hospital. I am glad that all the doctors, scientist, and companies made changes so were can all feel safe. If you have any allergies hay fever, sinus, eczema, and skin problems you might be sensitive to latex. So please if have reactions contact your doctor. I still have health problems like Asthma and I still deal with depression. It is a constant battle. When going to stores going around tires, shoes, sport equipment it is unbearable, I just hold my breath. I know it seem silly but I do this so I will not have a reaction. Driving around while the construction workers are putting down new roads and they use latex it is difficult breathing. In spite, of that we need knew roads and the Construction Workers work very hard to make sure that our roads are safe. We should all think of them when we see the new roads and look out for the Construction Workers so they can be safe while they are at work. I have been diagnosis with Asthma, Respiratory problems, and allergic to latex you may try to avoid these areas if possible. I do recognize that these construction workers work hard to make our streets safe. Because we need repairs on the roads and they just happens to use latex. Thanks to all the people that made changes in the medical field and food service so that everyone realizes this problem with latex was our entire problem.

One day I just happened to watch the Health channel, the discussion was concerns on Surgeons leaving instruments, sponges, gauzes, etc. in the patient after the operation was complete. A Surgeon is trying to change the procedures in the operating room. The Surgeon had a ideal, he said to himself if the grocery store can scan the food with a bar-code the purpose keeping track of stock and sales. Why can't it be done in the operating room to keep track of each item that is used in the operating procedures? The Surgeon stated that "we as Surgeons have deep concerns about our patients, we want to say to own patients yes the surgery went well." The Surgeon had the scan machine in the operating room and had each items for surgery labeled. The Nurse was scanning each item to prepare for surgery, and after surgery each item would be scanned to keep track of each items used in the operation procedures. The Surgeon was trying to make the operating room run more efficient. I don't know what stages that the Surgeon is in to complete his ideal.

Now I look at my life different, because of depression. I did not want to go to a Psychiatrist for therapy, but I had no choice. My life was dark, empty, I wanted to harm myself, and harm others. My World was not the same anymore. I was prescribed drugs and I did have some side effects. However, the drugs helped me slow down and look at my life. I was able to focus, and then while I focused I was able to help myself . I had to begin to heal and deal with the deep pain that was inside my heart and soul. I was in a place where hope, love, and peace did not exist. I was desperate and I felt alone. I thought this battle was only mind. I found out that many people were suffering the same battle.

ABOUT THE AUTHOR

Marion Ronee Daney have been writing poetry for years, and lives in Michigan. She is a single parent of her wonderful son, Jonathan. She knew deep inside her heart that her Heavenly Father gave her this precious gift of writing for a reason.

Marion Ronee Daney decided to return to school and take a Pharmacy Technician Program. She then worked in retail pharmacy for a couple of months and then in a hospital. After working in the hospital pharmacy for a couple of months, she noticed that after she wore the latex gloves when she did IV preparation. She would develop rashes on her hands.

A couple years went by, Marion noticed that while working in OR Pharmacy she started to itch all over her body and her nose constantly would run. The problem continued and worsened, she even ended up in ER.

Eventually, Marion was Disabled by the state of Michigan, because she had become Allergic to Latex. Her health problems are; Asthma and she went into a Deep Depression.

Marion realized that Destiny spoke to her and guided her to write this book," Latex Is Not My Friend." The NIGHTMARE that almost destroyed her, the Universe Graciously saved her with Wisdom and Love.

LaVergne, TN USA
05 March 2010
175127LV00001B/101/A